Praise for *Into the Soul of the World*

"As a far-flung journalist and celebrated editor, Brad Wetzler has led the very definition of an adventurous life, but in *Into the Soul of the World*, he gives an unflinching account of his interior adventures. Wetzler's soulful quest, by turns anguished and transcendent, will resonate with readers around the world who struggle to find purpose and a sense of the holy in the ambient jitter of the digital age."

—HAMPTON SIDES, author of *Ghost Soldiers*

"Reading Brad Wetzler's *Into the Soul of the World* is like embarking on a thrilling, dangerous journey—rivering straight into the heart of what matters most—to find yourself transformed. Ever the seeker, Wetzler wrestles with dark family secrets and triggered trauma, redefining what it means to be a man and spiritual being living in the twilight of our hyper-American materialism. If *Into the Soul of the World* belongs on a shelf next to *Eat, Pray, Love*, what lingers is Wetzler's relentless audacity to try to tell the truth, however uncomfortable—about families and lovers and our times—in hopes of setting himself, and us, free."

—MICHAEL PATERNITI, author of *Driving Mr. Albert*
and *The Telling Room*

"In the age of toxic masculinity, Brad Wetzler's *Into the Soul of the World* offers a powerful, profound, and deeply personal road map for actively cultivating a different kind of manhood. Through energetic and lively prose, Wetzler takes us inside the heart and mind of a man who refuses to conform to society's restrictive notion of manhood, and instead presents a new path for men to walk. This is not an easy path, Wetzler is clear, but we've never needed it more."

—EMILY RAPP BLACK, author of
The Still Point of the Turning World

"I've followed Brad Wetzler's travels around the globe with envy and admiration for more than two decades. He lived the dream. He also was living a lie, one that nearly destroyed him. *Into the Soul of the World* is his beautiful, terrifying, and witty travelogue, an essential chronicle of a life-saving journey into oneself."

—MARK ADAMS, author of *Tip of the Iceberg*

"*Into the Soul of the World* is a profound and profoundly moving meditation on one man's heroic quest to unchain himself from the tortured coils of childhood trauma. A guide as fearless as he is generous, Wetzler blazes a trail for all us anxious seekers through the promises and perils of psychiatry, drugs, Christianity, Buddhism, and yoga. A tale of heart-wrenching honesty and, ultimately, liberating compassion, this is a book that will change the lives of those yearning to find their own way back into the soul of the world."

—SARAH BIRD, author of *Last Dance on the Starlight Pier*

"Brad Wetzler is a born storyteller and a true seeker. His beautiful book reads like a trip to hell and back, with glimpses of paradise along the way. Wetzler's willing to climb the mountain, swim the river, crawl into the cave: whatever it takes to get some truth. As a result, *Into the Soul of the World* is an exhilarating read—the record of an extreme adventure and an unforgettable glimpse into the soul of a human being."

—CLINT WILLIS, author of *The Boys of Everest*

"*Into the Soul of the World* is full of an admirable power and urgency. It is not just a good, easy read, but a deep read as well. A part of the book's soul is how wide-ranging the story is in its exploration of trauma, bringing in not only psychology but an intelligent and sensitive telling of Wetzler's own life, along with many fascinating religious, spiritual, and philosophical excursions. At the center of the story is the failure of so much of medicalized psychology, making it a deeply relevant and important work to anyone interested in the state of psychotherapy today."

—DAVID GILBREATH BARTON, psychotherapist
and author of *Havel: Unfinished Revolution*

"After three decades of writing adventure stories, Brad Wetzler now delivers the ultimate adventure: a brave, big-hearted journey through trauma to self-transformation. For anyone and everyone faced with similar challenges, this is not just a book; it's a lamp to illuminate the rocky, painful, redemptive path forward."

—DANIEL COYLE, author of
The Talent Code and *The Culture Code*

into the soul
of the world

into the soul of the world

MY JOURNEY TO HEALING

BRAD WETZLER

hachette
BOOKS

NEW YORK

Hachette Go, an imprint of Hachette Books
Hachette Book Group
1290 Avenue of the Americas
New York, NY 10104
HachetteGo.com
Facebook.com/HachetteGo
Instagram.com/HachetteGo

First Edition: March 2023

Hachette Books is a division of Hachette Book Group, Inc.

The Hachette Go and Hachette Books name and logos are trademarks of Hachette Book Group, Inc.

The publisher is not responsible for websites (or their content) that are not owned by the publisher.

Print book interior design by Linda Mark.

Library of Congress Control Number: 2022950580

ISBNs: 978-0-306-82930-7 (hardcover); 978-0-306-82932-1 (ebook)

Printed in the United States of America

LSC-C

Printing 1, 2023

THIS BOOK IS MEMOIR. IT REFLECTS THE AUTHOR'S PRESENT recollections and perceptions of experiences over time. Some names and characteristics have been changed, some events have been compressed, and some dialogue has been re-created.

To my teachers,
formal and informal, past and present,
who have taught me how to live again.

You will not discover the limits of the soul by traveling, even if you wander over every conceivable path, so deep is its story.

—HERACLITUS, *Fragments*

How does it feel?

—BOB DYLAN, "Like a Rolling Stone"

Contents

Contents

Acknowledgments

SO MANY PEOPLE HAVE HELPED ME TO WRITE THIS BOOK ABOUT my journey to healing that I couldn't possibly name them all. Among them are wonderful friends who have helped me through conversation, caring acts, or the example of their lives. They include Matthew and Corinne Andrews, Joshua Home Edwards, Taylor White Moffitt, David Gilbreath Barton, Gillian and Mike Martin, Tamra Sattler, Amalia Var, Jim Cato, Benjy and Heather Wertheimer, David Newman, Brenda Mc-Morrow, and others. Abundant gratitude to the many talented, ethical professional healers I've been fortunate to work with, especially Susan Aposhyan, and the teachers at Yoga Pod Boulder; Practice Yoga of Austin, Texas; and CorePower Yoga of Boulder, Colorado.

Several wise and generous people either helped guide me through the publishing process, gave me feedback on the manuscript, or reminded me that the essence of good writing is to tell the truth and share from the heart, and pointed out when I fell short of that. They include Emily Rapp Black, Mark Adams, Greg Cliburn, Clint Willis, Skye Kerr Levy, Lisa Bennett, Victress Hitchcock, Mark Bryant, Laura Hohnhold, and others. Thank you to the older, more experienced editors I worked with at *Outside* magazine in the 1990s, especially Mark Bryant, Daniel Coyle, Hampton Sides, Laura Hohnhold, and Alex Heard, who taught me so much about the art and craft of telling stories in writing.

In the course of writing this book I have been supported, fed, and loved by Madeleine Tamayo Tilin.

I owe a great debt to my agent, Dan Milaschewski, of United Talent Agency, for nurturing this project.

Deep gratitude to Dan Ambrosio, my editor at Hachette Go. Without him this book would never have come into being.

Special thanks to Jack Kornfield, the late Ram Dass, Richard Freeman, Sharon Salzberg, and Tara Brach, wisdom teachers whom I've never met in person but whose books and recorded podcasts taught me so much during the past decade. Special thanks to Krishna Das, whose musical recordings and teachings kept me company during dark nights of the soul and whose chanting always brings me back to myself.

one

A MOUNTAIN OF A STORY

THE FIRST TIME I HEARD FROM OUR WRITER ON EVEREST AFTER the 1996 tragedy, I was seated at my desk, nibbling on a green chili breakfast burrito and reading the *New York Times* online. My computer's screen was filled with plane crashes and small wars in far-off nations. President Clinton grappled with gay people in the military.

My sunny, light-filled office on the second floor of *Outside* magazine's southwestern-themed building felt peaceful in comparison. It was just before 9 a.m. A cool morning breeze moved through my open balcony door—that clean mountain air. Across the street, I watched tourists posing for pictures next to an old train stop in the Santa Fe Railyard. Then the phone rang. I almost didn't pick up. Unless I was expecting a call, I rarely answered before nine.

I certainly wasn't expecting to hear that voice, which I recognized as soon as he spoke.

Today, author and journalist Jon Krakauer's first words still rattle around my head like lost dice. I would have known his efficient, clipped tone if he'd been speaking into one of those homemade toy phones made from two plastic cups linked by ten feet of kite string—or the distance of an ocean.

"Hey, Brad."

"Jon?" I gripped the phone tightly and pulled on the cord, trying to move it a few inches toward the door so I could take the call on the sunny balcony under the famous New Mexico sky, big and dotted with perfect-looking clouds, the mountains rising in the distance. I wanted to feel more connected—or at least less disconnected—to this writer who had just survived the deadliest day on the world's highest mountain while reporting a story for the magazine.

"Wait a second."

I was confused. The last I'd heard through Mark Bryant, the editor of *Outside*, my boss, and, in those days, Krakauer's editor and primary contact on all his stories for the magazine, our writer had made it safely back to base camp after a fast-moving blizzard pounded the granite peak on a day when dozens were descending from the summit. The storm had caught the climbers off guard. Some never made it off the summit ridge while others hurried toward their campsite down dangerous slopes in whiteout conditions. Some climbers made it back to their tents. But others become confused and lost and froze to death or fell off the mountain's steep slope. Eleven climbers were either dead or missing and presumed dead. We editors eventually learned that Jon had made it safely back to his tent, and a few days later, we learned that he had arrived back at base camp. From there, we thought he'd have to trek back out to civilization. So, we weren't expecting to hear from him for more than a week. Which is why I was confused, and overwhelmed, but more than anything else, relieved to hear his voice. He was alive.

"I'm in Kathmandu. I'm at a hotel."

He then explained that instead of trekking back out he and the other climbers had been picked up by a helicopter at Pheriche, a village with a small hospital about eight miles from Everest base camp.

"Fucking A, Jon. I can't tell you how glad I am to hear your voice. I know this is a stupid question, but are you okay?" It was the only question I could think to ask.

I tried to picture the best-selling author of *Into the Wild*, a consummate adventure writer, and a longtime contributor to our magazine, in the aftermath of what he'd just gone through. Of course, I had zero ability to relate to the traumas he'd experienced. I'd sat on my ass in a climate-controlled office for the past eight weeks worrying while he'd bled and suffered in more ways than I could comprehend.

I listened as he filled me in on a few details of the scene on the mountain after the storm and the conditions of some of the climbers with whom I was familiar.

"Fuck," I said.

As I spoke, I felt a wave of emotion and even fought back a tear.

Why? I'm not sure. I didn't know Krakauer. We had spoken only a handful of times, primarily during the six months before the climb when I was working the phones to try to land him on a commercial guided climbing team. Moreover, I and the other editors bore no responsibility for his safety, and none of us could take any credit for his success on the mountain. The idea to climb to the summit of Mount Everest had been a thousand-percent his. As Mark recently told me: "Our idea was to have somebody of Krakauer's credibility cover Everest's growing commercialism from base camp. We certainly didn't aspire to put one of our writers' lives at risk by going to the top."

Furthermore, we editors hadn't done an ounce of the real work. We hadn't put ourselves in exceedingly dangerous places. Nor had we suffered a whit. And yet . . . I was flooded with emotions, and even today I'm not sure why. I guess it was because I had expended significant emotional capital worrying about him. All of us editors had. And this: on some barely conscious level, I, a thirty-year-old associate editor who was taking this call from Krakauer because Mark wasn't available, suspected that the climbers who survived that brutal storm on Mount Everest on May 10, 1996, would have a difficult time healing from the trauma and finding peace. If ever they did.

But this moment wasn't about me. This phone call, this magazine story. None of it was about me. Though I admit: I have often lost sight of this reality.

We continued talking for another few minutes. He told me a little about what he'd been through, and then he said he had plans to start writing very soon after he returned to Seattle.

"No, no, I spoke with Mark about this. He said to tell you that you can take all the time you need. I mean, you could wait a year to write this story. We don't care. Just get home and get rested and recovered. We can talk in a few weeks or longer."

"Do you know if Mark's around?" Jon usually consulted only with Mark.

"I haven't seen him."

I looked down at the project management folder that contained nearly two years of notes, clipped articles, and correspondence from guiding companies, and became lost in thought. Since my first days as an intern at the magazine, I had been an armchair Everest buff, reading books, watching videos, and keeping tabs on each climbing season. Why? I'm not sure I know. This is just what I do. I become obsessed; I go down rabbit holes. Eventually, I got promoted to assistant editor and became the maven of the magazine's adventure beat. I began keeping a file about Everest. Soon my file grew thick with articles and written notes from my interviews with various Everest experts. Some of these experts kept telling me that we editors should send a writer to Everest to write about the rise of commercially guided expeditions. Several new outfits were advertising their services and promising potential clients they'd do the hard work of setting ropes, carrying heavy gear, making camp, calling the tactical shots—practically everything except the actual climbing. The cost to the client: $65,000.

Eventually, during the winter of 1993–1994, I wrote a story pitch in which I'd argued that we should get a writer to base camp sooner than later: "Eventually, the shit will hit the fan," I stated. I delivered the pitch in an editorial meeting in the conference room of our offices then located in downtown Chicago. At the end of the pitch, I suggested we consider both mountaineering writer Greg Child and Jon Krakauer as potential writers.

That far tamer Everest story was largely forgotten. It never happened. But I remained vitally interested in all things Everest. We did offer it to Krakauer in March 1995, but he turned it down. And then he surprised us all when later he called Mark and said that he *would* go to Everest if we got him on a team and that he wanted to try to climb to the top.

I was beyond thrilled when I heard this. This was even better. Practically all of us at the magazine began working toward making this story happen. And Mark was kind enough to anoint me chief shepherd of the nascent project. Thus, Krakauer called me when he couldn't track Mark down.

I must have spaced out ten seconds. When I drifted back to reality, Krakauer was ready to get off the phone. "Gotta go, Brad."

"Okay, well. Take it easy on yourself. You've been through a lot." As if this seasoned mountaineer and journalist needed life advice from me.

THUS BEGAN THE FINAL CHAPTER OF MY SIX-YEAR CAREER AS AN UP-and-coming editor at one of the nation's most respected, award-winning magazines. In my work as editorial project manager of the Everest story, I had primarily made a lot of phone calls. I'd helped get Krakauer a place on a premiere mountain guiding company. Other than that, I'd prayed a lot for his safe return. But today, when I look back on the spring and summer of 1996, I can see that I got pretty jacked up on raw exuberance. I also became poisoned by my own inner grandiosity. In my head, I was already writing my own press releases. I believed my involvement in this Everest story would help me fulfill my dream of becoming an adventure writer myself. As the summer wore on, I shepherded Krakauer's story through the editorial process at *Outside*. I reviewed the manuscript when it landed on my desk, oversaw the team of fact-checkers and the creation of the two-page graphic sidebar. I found myself being interviewed on camera for ABC News at Mark's request. A month later, Mark promoted me to senior editor. And after the story appeared on newsstands in the September 1996 issue of *Outside* with bold lettering that read "The Story on Everest," I sat for dozens more radio, TV, and newspaper interviews. I began receiving phone calls from editors of other magazines offering me writing assignments for adventure-related stories. I had it all figured out;

it had never been my goal to become a great *editor* of adventure stories; my goal was to be the adventure *writer* himself.

In early November, about three months after "Into Thin Air" appeared on newsstands, I gave Mark my notice, packed my *Outside* office into boxes, thanked my boss and the rest of the staff, and set up a home office in the new house I shared with Di, my wife. If now wasn't the perfect time to make my break and step into the life of my dreams, full of adventurous travel to exotic places, when would the right time be? In this moment, becoming a great adventure writer felt like more than just a dream—it felt, excuse the hyperbole, like my destiny.

It all sounds so logical and reasonable now. As I organized my new home office, there was one memo I didn't get or at least didn't read. If only I'd spent more time studying the writings of Freud and Jung, or at least just looked up the word *destiny*. If I had, I might have learned that destiny, it turns out, is a future scenario, one's destination. We can dream about our destiny, the place we'd like to end up. But we cannot escape our fate, a word I should also have looked up, something a tad more twisted and dark. Fate is what the universe has planned for us, and its synonym, somewhat appropriately, is *doom*. If becoming a successful adventure writer was my destiny, then losing everything—my wife, my house, my money, my career, my sanity, and nearly my life within ten years of the publication of "Into Thin Air"—was my fate.

I never could have imagined that within that decade, due to undiagnosed, untreated PTSD and complex PTSD, I would be brought to my knees by visually graphic and other times purely emotion-driven flashbacks. I would end up too depressed to carry on and numbed out on a massive cocktail of twenty-three psychotropic pills per day. I could never have anticipated that I would become a housebound zombie, living off government disability checks, or that, much later, I'd try to pull my life together by reimagining myself as a spiritual seeker on the road to redemption across the Holy Land. I certainly never could have predicted that I'd temporarily abandon my writing career to become a headband-wearing yoga teacher. Or that I'd be twice divorced and endure the Mother of All Midlife Crises.

How could I have foreseen that I would one day kneel at the feet of a hundred-year-old yogi in a cave in the Himalayas and that he'd bless me by literally smacking me on the head, leading to a twelve-hour mystical experience during which the curtain of the universe was pulled back for me, and I saw the unification of All?

As I sat in my office the day of that call, I thought I was building the foundation for a solid career as a journalist and travel writer. Who knew where that could lead, but lectures, books, fame, and material wealth were certainly my hoped-for destiny. I had no idea that I was a broken man, doomed to external adventures that were humbling and humiliating, as well as a man fated for a decade of challenging inner work needed to heal and finally make sense of my life.

All of this happened to me.

And I'm still here to tell the story.

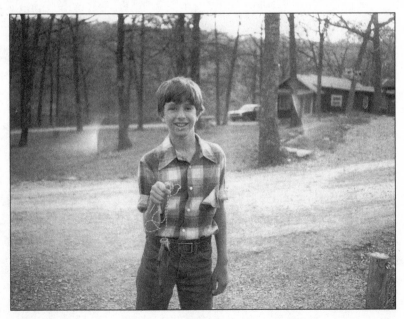

I caught this fish, my first, during a grade school field trip to a farm in Kansas.

two

THE RIVER (IS EVERYWHERE)

EVERY ADVENTURE WRITER WORTH HIS SALT KNOWS THAT A story evolves over time. You don't set out knowing exactly where to begin. You must first hack at it, bully it, move through it, play with it. You must fight your way through the messy middle. You must bring forth the crisis, the climax, the resolution, all of it, and then you must write the ending. Or take your first stab at the ending. Then and only then do you have the clarity of mind to see a story's true beginning.

So, fuck fate. Fuck doom. Fuck hubris, and fuck Icarus, too. Maybe I did leave the starting gate too fast and hard. But this story is not about those themes. It's not about Everest or Jon Krakauer either.

This story is about faith. It's also about other words—adventure, trauma, addiction, and how we humans heal. But I argue that faith is inherent in all of it.

And so, the story's truest beginning is this:

May 1978, and I was twelve years old. The morning fog was lifting on the sandy bank of Arkansas's White River. I climbed into an aluminum canoe and carefully walked to the seat at the bow. I lifted the plastic paddle and held it in my hand, feeling the weight of the blade and the texture of the ridged grip. I felt anxious, even queasy, remembering the grim face of a visitor at our campsite the previous evening. "It's rained nonstop for over a week," he warned. "This on top of a very wet spring. The river is too high to run right now. I can give you your money back, and you can stay at a hotel in town. Last weekend, three parties wrapped their canoes around trees, bent in half. They barely made it out alive."

Or was I more disturbed by the near unanimous reaction of the fathers who stood listening? One voiced what all seemed to be thinking: "Thank you for your advice, but we've come too far not to run. We will be fine." I felt so anxious after this that I barely slept. And now my stomach fluttered, and my limbs buzzed with anxiety. I glanced over my shoulder and watched my dad step into the canoe and sit at the stern. Handsome, six feet tall, imposing. Throughout my life, I watched as strangers asked him whether he was Mario Andretti or Senator Gary Hart. A lawyer with a big, politically connected law firm in suburban Kansas City, he spoke with certainty about how the world worked, how business worked, how life worked. I noticed that a lot of younger, less successful men looked up to him. But over time, I also noticed that he looked down on many of the men who worshipped him.

We pushed off. The canoe glided away from the shore toward the river's main channel. The current grabbed the narrow, aluminum boat and began to push us downriver sideways, and I heard my dad voice his frustration.

"God darn it. Paddle, Brad."

I was paddling.

The next thirty seconds were, in retrospect, comical, although they didn't feel that way at the time. My dad, whom I'd only been in a canoe with once before, struggled to control our direction. We floated sideways, and then we swung akimbo and slightly backward, before our boat corrected and we headed downstream. I looked back at the sandbar where the other fathers and sons were laughing at us. Not that they were any better. Just about every canoe before and after us did the same thing.

As our boat straightened out, my father reminded me of something that he'd said four or five times already that morning.

"You are the power, Brad. If you don't paddle hard, I can't steer us."

"Okay, okay."

I dug my blade into the river and paddled hard. Years later, when I worked as a camp counselor in Maine and learned how to paddle a canoe solo, I learned that my dad's adage was incorrect. The person in the stern must know how to steer a canoe on their own, regardless of how hard the kid in front is paddling.

But on that day, I focused on paddling hard. It was my job, and I was an earnest kid, and I intended to do it well. And, like any kid, I wanted to make my father proud.

We spent the morning canoeing like Laurel and Hardy. We entered rapids sideways, backward, always to the refrain, "You're not paddling hard enough."

By noon, I was beginning to catch on. I *was* paddling hard enough. Was it possible that my dad didn't know what he was doing? But I didn't dare say that. So I kept paddling and kept assuring him I was paddling hard.

We stopped on a sandbar for lunch, and then we launched our canoe again. We came to a downed tree that had fallen during the spring heavy rains. We portaged around it and then set the canoe back in the water and pushed off again. As we had in the morning, we entered the channel going sideways. Only at this place, the river was running faster and deeper.

"Paddle harder, Brad. You're not giving me the power I need to steer the boat."

I dug in harder and pulled the paddle back and through.

But we kept going sideways. The current lifted the right side of the canoe, gravity pulled it back down, and water poured over the side, first slowly, then rapidly. Before I could take a breath, the current dumped us over. I felt my balls constrict into my abdomen, and I couldn't catch my breath. And then, eventually, my body got used to the cold water. As I floated downstream, I felt weightless. My dad drifted toward the bank. I spotted him crawling out of the water on his hands and knees. But I kept drifting farther away from the banks. I felt free.

Then I felt a massive jerk and my head plunged underwater. I feared I would drown right then and there. But then my head surfaced. I took a massive, gasping inhale only to be plunged under the water once again. *Okay, now I am going to die*, I thought. But again, my head surfaced, and this time it stayed above water. I was terribly confused. I tried to look behind me, but my life jacket was in the way. I felt something hard against my torso. I touched it with my hand—a tree, with sharp, broken branches. I put two and two together and concluded that my lifejacket had snagged on a submerged log. I was stuck and I was in pain. The current pressed my skinny, twelve-year-old body into the log, and at the same time it clawed at me, begging me to be free. I looked over at my father. He stood on the bank, motionless, staring back at me.

I felt calm. *Why?* I wondered. I felt out of time, as if I were watching myself stranded on a log in a parallel universe.

I spent the next few minutes in this Zen-like state. Then I began to feel again—fear and frustration. I looked down at my father. He was still on the bank. *Aren't you going to do something?* He seemed incapable of movement, entirely stuck in his own fear. I hope that's what was happening for him. The alternative, that he chose not to rescue his son, would be too difficult to comprehend.

A FEW MORE MINUTES MUST HAVE PASSED. FEAR TURNED TO RAGE. I looked up at the sky and pleaded with God to save me. Nothing. Of course, God wasn't going to save me: he didn't save his own son when he was dying on the cross. I felt the log shift underneath me. I feared I would be pulled under again. Then I was, eyes and mouth sealed shut, arms flailing, grabbing, to no avail. And suddenly, thankfully, I could breathe and see again. But I was still stuck. *Where's my dad? Is he getting help?* I felt lost and hopeless. Trapped. Abandoned. Utterly alone. Totally fucked.

Thirty-three years later, I can see and feel everything as clearly as when it happened. The memories have not faded with time. I hear the clunk of a canoe striking the log and the back of my head. I feel a blunt strike against my shoulders and neck. I hear my friend Bill's dad shouting. I see his arm reach for me but miss. And then, I am free. I feel free. Freer than I've felt before. My head hurt. My side hurt, and I later noticed cuts and bruises that lasted a week. But none of that mattered, because I was free, floating down the river, suspended and somehow safe.

Today I believe I understand what my father really meant when he said, "You are the power": *I have zero idea what I'm doing in this here canoe. I don't know how to steer. I don't know how to read a raging river. So, kiddo, it's up to you. Oh, and guess what, son? If we tip over, it will be your fault.*

Ron Morris, our group's leader, scooped me up and set me in the bottom of a boat, where I lay crying. And then I heard my father's voice: "Get up, son. You're fine."

And on one level he was correct. I'd only suffered cuts and bruises—albeit deep bruises that ached for a week as I tried to focus on my seventh-grade classes at school—but I was definitely not fine. And there's a real way in which I would never be fine from that day forward.

That evening, while our exhausted group of boys and fathers sat around a campfire, our leader, Ron Morris, led us in a prayer of thanks to Jesus for saving me from drowning. I stared into the flames, tears welling in my eyes. I didn't feel fine. I never felt at home in nature again. I never felt at home in my own body again. Freud wrote that we will unconsciously gravitate toward the very things that wounded us. We try and try and try to have a better experience. I became an adventure-travel writer, even though I had a difficult relationship with nature. I tried to outrun myself, my own body. Looking back, it was all a big cosmic setup. I put myself in situations that would traumatize me as an unconscious attempt to heal. I found myself stranded in remote campsites in roadless regions. Or on planes to far-off places in nature where I would have little control over outcomes. Trauma was layered up on trauma. And that's when I turned to a psychiatrist. Unfortunately, this one had a penchant and a reputation for overmedicating his clients. I took pill after pill until I was taking more than twenty tablets and capsules per day and barely left my own house.

The last thing I want to do is throw my father under the bus in my story. Even from where I sit, I can acknowledge that he's not a bad man, although he does have a difficult relationship with the truth. And today, despite many requests for a conversation about our shared history, we have never resolved our disparate experiences and memories about that day on the river. But the lie that hurt me most came the night we returned home from the canoe trip. I ran toward my mother to tell her about my ordeal on the submerged log—those minutes of feeling trapped, as if I might die.

"Honey, Brad's exaggerating. Nothing like that happened. His shirt got snagged on a twig."

My shirt got snagged on a twig. I knew that wasn't true. And if that had been the case, why didn't Dad bother to saunter out into the placid waters and unhook said shirt? "Your shirt got snagged" became his mantra about that canoe trip for the next forty years. A decade later, I received confirmation of my inner reality when I ran into Ron Morris at a Kansas City Royals baseball game and he told me how terrified he'd been watching the near-drowning from his boat many yards downstream.

I knew my father's version of reality wasn't true, but I never said it. He was my dad. And I didn't want to embarrass him. I loved him. I still do.

AFTER THAT DAY, I STILL LOVED MY FATHER AS DEEPLY AS ANY SON does. But the seeds of confusion and later rage had been planted. Because I also saw my father as a hypocrite and a liar. He seemed to need to curate, even control, my reality. As I developed my own ideas about the world, tensions between us rose. If protested, he reacted with sarcastic, cutting put-downs, glares, or by ignoring me. He seemed to give my siblings tacit consent to treat me like this, too. Should I comply with my reality or his became a near-constant question to my young, vulnerable mind. Eventually, my image of him was split into two distinct fathers: one version was idealistic, my dad as the do-no-wrong holy father. The other?

The opposite: a cruel, manipulative, uncaring motherfucker. How does a child—or, later, that adult—reconcile this psychic split? You become a seeker, an achiever, and you set your sights on setting the world on fire with your own grandiose sense of genius.

After that canoeing accident, my father never seemed the same. I can't say for certain that the accident had anything to do with what I experienced as his shift in behavior. But he seemed markedly different. Perhaps my perceptions opened. He regularly came to dinner drunk on Gallo and slurring his speech. Often, after dinner, he drank gin until he passed out and could not be roused. Many times the rest of my family split when he did this, my brother to his girlfriends, my mother to Junior League meetings or to help my sister with her homework. Me? I couldn't leave his side. On a dozen or more occasions, as the credits to the *Tonight Show* rolled and Doc Severinsen's trumpet wailed, I'd grab his arm and pull him out of his recliner. My arm around his shoulder like a big brother, I'd walk him to bed.

Once, on a camping trip in Colorado, he marched my older brother and me into the backcountry. The three of us fumbled to cook a freeze-dried stroganoff dish in the rain. By dusk, he'd drunk enough gin to need to lie down alone in the tent. My brother and I stayed up talking under the brilliant Perseid meteor showers. I came to bed last. I tried to nudge him to say good night, but he didn't budge. His mouth was propped open, and his tongue hung out sloppily. For a split second, my heart sunk into my belly. I thought he was dead.

Decades later, in my early fifties, I would be told independently by a psychiatrist and therapist that, in their assessment, I had suffered abuse and neglect during my childhood. But that didn't help the young boy struggling to build his identity and place in the world. Throughout my adolescence, when I could, I fell asleep listening to talk radio or reading about Jesus in the New Testament. I found solace in the actions and ideas of this radical man from Galilee, this free spirit, this believer in justice. A sense of righteousness and maybe temporary okayness. I grew to loathe the mornings after as much as the late nights. I would eat my

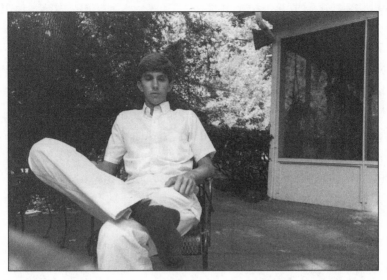

During my teens in the Kansas City suburbs the depressions grew deep and frequent.

cereal and watch the *Today Show*. When my dad entered the breakfast nook dressed in his pin-striped suit and reeking of cologne, ready for his day of lawyering, I cringed. And when he tried to father me or otherwise tell me how *to be a man,* I raged silently. I was a skinny, lonely preteen suffering from anorexia, insomnia, and depression, but I was hopped up on Jesus stories, and I was pissed off. If only I were brave enough, I'd have toppled the breakfast table and shaken my fist at him and driven him out of the temple of my life.

But I was a boy. And he was my father.

In high school, when he moved out, back in, out again, and then back in just for Christmas Eve and Day and ordered us all to put on a show for his mother and talk to her as if he lived in the house when in fact he had lived across town, I walked the nearby creek and raised my fist to the steely Kansas winter sky. I felt possessed by pure, unadulterated, high-test anger—far more anger than my six-foot, 125-pound body could reasonably house. And I couldn't mention a word to my mom or dad about how wrong and hypocritical this faux Christmas felt. They would deflect it. "Brad, you're just too angry of a person," my dad will still tell me on the rare occasions that we talk. "What happened to the sweet, fun kid you used to be?"

And today, as far as I know, nobody, not my mother, not my brother or sister, ever said a word to him about any of this. But I have. I remember.

A child will twist his own mind into knots to protect his image of a parent as caring, loving, committed. It never occurs to a child that a parent doesn't have his best interest in mind. Why won't a child speak his mind to a neglectful parent? Easy: he fears losing his sacred bond. He knows, on some deep level, that the cost of rebelling is abandonment, and no child will take the risk of that loss.

And so, as a child, I said nothing. And when I was a teenager and did say something, I was criticized for being angry and disrespectful.

Over the years, I came to see myself as toxic. I believed I was the problem. How could it be anybody else's fault but mine? I was too smart-alecky. Too disrespectful. Too this or that. Too everything. But also, never enough.

And that happy-go-lucky, people-pleasing junior editor at the high-profile adventure magazine, who commissioned and edited famous, successful stories was still holding all that anger inside, trapped, with nowhere to go. Whether I was editing, writing, or hiking with Di, I spent an extraordinary amount of energy holding my own darkness at bay, to maintain the smile on my face. With each passing year, these tasks grew more and more Herculean.

I've learned volumes about trauma and its effects. We can withstand many of life's traumas if we have supportive people to talk to. According to the prevailing theory, trauma gets stuck in the body. Talking about the traumatic events, processing them in a supportive community, is how we heal, as attested to by van der Kolk, Susan Aposhyan, Peter Levine, and many others.

Healing childhood trauma is more difficult and complex because the child's brain is not yet developed. And most children don't have an adult nearby who is wise and supportive enough to help. On their own, a child will try to think his way out of the trauma, and that's a task no child is up to. His mind can end up resembling a piece of twine that's become hopelessly knotted and tangled. The child, and later the adult, will make twisted assumptions about himself, about the world, about life. He will blame himself for the events that caused the trauma. Ultimately, he will disconnect from himself and suffer from depression, dissociation, anxiety, insomnia, negative self-talk, and low self-esteem. Trauma specialists now believe that the experience doesn't need to be a dramatic, life-endangering accident to cause post-traumatic stress disorder or PTSD.

Growing up in a dysfunctional family can cause relational or attachment trauma and lead to complex PTSD symptoms. In a dysfunctional family marked by emotional abuse or neglect, as I have come to view my family, a child is often scapegoated. The family, overtly and covertly, blames a child for their problems as a means of deflecting attention from the real problems. Instead of a single traumatic event, a child in this role might experience a continual barrage of subtle attacks on his worthiness, sense of belonging, and even his very identity. These attacks might come in the form of gaslighting, verbal abuse, and other obvious forms of manipulation. But they also can come in the form of thousands upon thousands of subtle negative facial expressions and sarcastic put-downs over years or decades. The family's intent, whether conscious or unconscious, is to make the child feel like an Other, like he cannot be his authentic self and still remain a member of the family, like he is not part of the pack. After all, we are pack animals. Indeed, by adulthood, he feels toxic, broken, and like an outsider in his own family, in his own body, in his own life. This unease carries into adult relationships with partners, colleagues, and bosses. His fear of rejection and unconscious behavior may turn his new friend groups or places of employment into his old family of origin, where the cycle of scapegoating continues.

Today, when I meet a teenager who seems obsessed with keeping adults happy, I cringe inside. I want to call 911.

three

FALLING IN LOVE WITH ADVENTURE

ARRIVED SMILING AT OUTSIDE'S OFFICES IN DOWNTOWN CHI-cago on a snowy mid-December morning in 1990. The previous Friday I'd wrapped up work on my master's degree at Northwestern University's prestigious Medill School of Journalism. I stomped the snow off my boots and checked in with the receptionist, who led me to a cubicle against a mauve-tinted window overlooking Chicago's tony Gold Coast. I hung my coat and sat at my new desk and opened the *New York Times*. When the other intern arrived, a bearded fellow my age named Alex, I introduced myself, and he explained the ins and outs of my new job.

"Basically, we type. We receive manuscripts from our writers in the mail, and you retype the stories into the computer so it's in our system. Then you print the story out, and you distribute it to the editors assigned to it."

Alex handed me an envelope. I opened it and took out the typed manuscript it contained. And I got to work. I typed. Hard and fast. I was a longtime reader of *Outside*, dating back to high school, and had many times imagined working there as an editor, maybe an adventure writer. Right now, my job was to type manuscripts, and I was determined to be the best intern they'd ever seen.

Beth, the managing editor, must have thought very highly of my typing, because after three months working, I was summoned to her office and offered a full-time position. My title: editorial assistant. My salary: $18,000 a year or, after taxes, biweekly payments of $500. My main responsibility was fact-checking the magazine's Gear and Travel departments. I was thrilled. This was literally a dream come true.

In the 1990s, *Outside* was one of the most successful magazines in the country. It was thick with advertising from Nike, the major auto companies, and outdoor brands such as The North Face. And its readership consisted largely of successful, moneyed, weekend warrior types. I seemed to fit in well, too, as the magazine was staffed by twenty- and thirtysomethings who were smart, funny, and loaded with white privilege. We hailed from good schools and presumably decent families. I looked up to my peers. I could tell that the editors were more than just colleagues. We seemed to care about each other. We were drinking buddies, and on weekends, we went mountain biking at state parks or attended Cubs games at Wrigley Field. I was barely three months out of grad school and only twenty-five years old, but I'd already landed my dream job.

Looking back, I realize I barely knew who I was, even as I stepped enthusiastically into this new role, this new identity, this new life. Born and raised in a suburb of Kansas City, I was tall and lanky, with a mop of brown hair that I parted on the side like a TV weatherman. Like a weatherman, I smiled often and was eager to please—too eager. But I loved my new job. I was earnest, too. I worked hard. I arrived each morning thirty minutes early, wielding a Starbucks coffee, a blueberry muffin, and the *New York Times*. As if I were setting a table for a king, I spread the newspaper of record across my desk, and then, sipping and munching, I devoured the paper section by section. When I reached the back page, I turned to the magazines that were delivered to our office: *Surfer, Backpacker, Bicycling, Ski and Skiing, Sports Illustrated, Climbing, Rock and Ice*. And then I surfed the web (which took longer then) for news about explorers and adventurers who risked their lives trying to climb tall

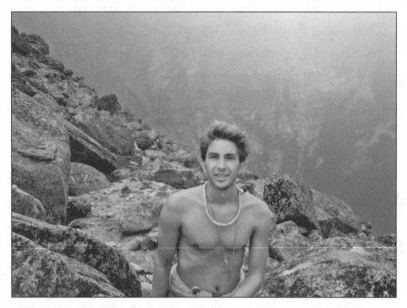

In the late 1980s, I worked as a "trip leader" guiding groups of fifteen-year-olds to the top of Maine's Mount Katahdin and other New England peaks.

mountains, surf big waves, pull sleds to the North and South Pole, hack their way through dense tropical jungles, on and on and on.

I loved my job because I worked for a magazine that published stories about humans living inspired, adventurous lives, lives that said fuck you to a traditional nine-to-five job and focused on adventure and travel instead. For a twenty-five-year-old man or woman, what wasn't to like about it? If a subject we wanted to write about didn't quite fit with our mission, we made it fit. (One of *Outside*'s most-loved articles of all time was "King of the Ferretleggers," about English miner Reg Mellor's wacky hobby of stuffing live ferrets down his pants to see if he could bear the painful consequences.) In truth, the world was our oyster.

I loved stories. I loved words. Editing and writing adventure stories suited me and my own creative, storytelling brain. Adventuring, albeit a far lighter variety than high-altitude mountaineering, was right up my alley, too. Though I'd grown up in the dull, flat state of Kansas, I soon realized I was one of the most experienced outdoorspeople on staff. As a boy, I'd gone on hiking and ski vacations in the Colorado Rockies. In college, I'd worked as a trip leader at a summer camp in Maine, guiding teenaged boys on weeklong backpacking trips across New England's highest peaks, including New Hampshire's Mount Washington and Maine's Mount Katahdin. Back in those days, I had a 1970s-era VW bus I drove across the United States more than once. And while studying philosophy at King's College in London, I spent several weeks hitchhiking across England, Wales, and Ireland. After college, I worked as a ski lift operator (until I seriously blew out my knee and retreated to Kansas to rehab it). All this experience in the wild and on the road served me well when it came to writing and editing stories for *Outside*.

I didn't just love the work—I loved the people I worked with, which was a good thing, as the hours were long, sometimes more than fifty per week. In the early 1990s, my life could be boiled down to working at "the magazine" and exploring Chicago with Dianna, a smart, charming, and warmhearted graduate of the University of Michigan I met in graduate school at Northwestern and the woman I'd later marry.

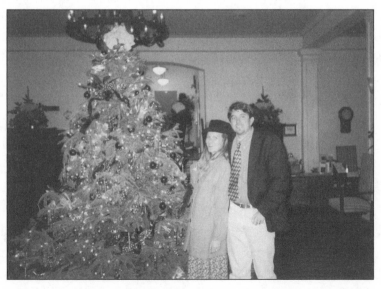

A stranger took this picture of Di and me celebrating our wedding night in Santa Fe, New Mexico, in December of 1994.

There was no formal training to become a great editor. We learned on the fly, by doing—the old "baptism by fire" approach. I must have shown promise to the higher-ups, because over the next year, in addition to fact-checking, I was fed a steady stream of new, increasingly complex projects. I even landed an assignment to write my first travel story, about fly fishing in the Missouri Ozarks at my dad's favorite spot. I even invited him to come with me. Next, I wrote a news article about a new bear repellant consisting of cayenne pepper spray. I followed that with an investigative feature about corruption at the US Forest Service. If you could graph my career trajectory at that time, it would look like a rocket's, headed for the stratosphere. In the fall of 1992, I was promoted to assistant editor, and then, eighteen months later, associate editor. Soon I had an office on the main hallway, kitty-corner from Mark's. I was helping manage the news section and assigning and editing features. I was on my way to the top, and I was enjoying every minute of it.

Outside was killing it, too. The magazine reached more than a million readers per month. Our stories and authors were frequently featured on the evening news and the *Today Show*. One page of advertising went for tens of thousands of dollars, and as advertising revenue grew, so did the magazine; the fall issues then were fat as books. *Outside* was even starting a television channel. The editors were young and bold, and we believed in what we were doing. When we'd had a few beers, we compared our influence on the zeitgeist to the *Rolling Stone* of the 1970s and the *New Yorker* under Tina Brown. I wasn't the only one who felt as if I was taking off to the stratosphere—we all did. I made my home in a studio apartment on a tree-lined street in Lincoln Park, two blocks from Dianna's.

We never know how we are seen by others. But if you asked one of my workmates then, I suspect they would have told you I was a smart, funny, talented, optimistic young man. A pleasant, hardworking midwesterner, with a touch of quirk. While others rode top-of-the-line ten-speeds they bought on a company discount, I boasted about my old one-speed, painted gold and purchased for five dollars at a garage sale, that I called Golden Boy. I seriously doubt anybody suspected that my outside veneer and how I felt inside were at serious odds. Nobody would have described me then as depressed, angry, or prickly. That would come later. Back then, I was like my mother: I liked to smile, and I liked it when other people were happy with me. Looking back, I didn't really know myself very well at all. I was simply playing a part.

At the time, I was concerned only with building a career, a life, a name for myself, and money in the bank was nice too. I gave no attention or thought to issues such as personal development. I was unaware of the dangers of believing one's own press. As Carl Jung wrote, in our twenties and thirties, we are consumed with building a persona:

> The persona is a complicated system of relations between individual consciousness and society . . . a kind of mask, designed on the one hand to make a definite impression upon others, and, on the other, to conceal the true nature of the individual.
>
> There's nothing wrong with the persona, it's a normal stage of development between the person and society.

Trouble happens, however, if we move into midlife and still *identify* with that persona—that is, if we come to believe that our mask is the whole story. Eventually, the persona, the mask created in the first half of life, must fall off if we are to stay connected to our true self. This process of letting go of our false self can be painful, messy, but it's necessary. In this country, where materialism and denial of aging and death are so common, a man will resist this transformation at his own peril. Instead of real change, this man will dye his gray hair, buy a fast red car, and put a much younger woman in the passenger seat. And wake up ten years later still a man-child obsessed with career titles, material wealth, and power.

I tried to take the other route. I listened to Jung when he wrote, in midlife, all of life's problems have spiritual answers. The results? Read on.

four

THE STRANGER

ONE DAY, IN 1992, A STRANGER, A BEARDED MAN WEARING A pink oxford shirt and blue jeans skulked past my office and disappeared into Mark's. An hour or so later, I heard Mark and the stranger talking in the hallway. Other editors had joined them. I stopped stuffing rejection letters into envelopes and listened. The stranger was telling a story about a recent ascent of a difficult, remote peak in Patagonia. *Wait, is that who I think it is?* I couldn't stand it any longer. I stood up and walked to the doorway, casually grabbing the door frame above me, trying to appear more confident than I was.

The stranger continued with a precise account of the climb. I don't remember his exact words. My mind disconnected from the present moment, and my imagination filled in the blanks.

I heard an editor say, "Wow," and my attention swung back to the physical realm.

"This is going to be a great story, Jon," a different editor said. The voice belonged to Donovan, who seemed to be our own literary shooting star. A senior editor from Chicago, Donovan was already writing feature stories for the *New Yorker*. Smart, bombastic, and kind, he seemed to write exclusively about the biggest and most intense topics, and he always had a nugget of storytelling wisdom to share with us junior editors. "You've got to make the box before you break the box," he liked to say about setting up the story with a strong argument before you begin to deconstruct it. He was the archetype of the adventure writer. Long hair, John Lennon glasses, tall, handsome. Brave. I only knew him during nine-to-five hours, but he seemed to have the world by its tail.

Eventually, I couldn't stand being unseen and unheard. I moved into the hallway.

"Buck! Meet Jon. Jon, meet Buck. Well, that's what we call him. This is Brad."

Mark rested his hand on my shoulder. As a kid, my brother called me Bucky because my front teeth stuck out. But braces fixed that. And at some point, friends caught on and shortened my nickname to Buck. Buck. I liked it better than Bucky. It was more . . . adult. Buck was the dog in Jack London's *Call of the Wild*. To me, the moniker suggested a strength, bravery. I never asked anybody to call me Buck, but I didn't mind it one bit. And while I didn't see myself as heroic, strong, or particularly brave, I believed I would deserve such a nickname once I became a bona fide adventure writer myself.

I shook the stranger's hand. It was firm. I looked down at his muscled forearms, revealed by his rolled-up sleeves. I had spoken to him as a fact-checker. I'd read all his feature stories, climbing adventures around the world. We were different. He was compact, intense, organized, forceful. I was easygoing, creative, intense in my own way, but always aiming to please. He didn't look like he needed or wanted to please anyone. That impressed me, and I tucked the observation away.

I stood and listened to the older editors banter. I soaked it all in. Someday, I hoped I would return to the halls of *Outside* and editors would swarm around me. Today, I see it. I was caught up in my own striving and desire for fame. Decades later, I'd have to face and try to heal my grandiose ideas about who I was. But at that time, I wanted to be an adventure writer, too. I wanted a life of adventure and maybe fame and fortune. And yet I hadn't a clue about who I really was.

We knocked off work early, and all the editors went out for beers at a dark bar with striped upholstery and smoky air. We all told stories. Stories were the currency around there.

The story I told everyone that night over my pint of lager, and a story I still tell on occasion, was about the time I hitchhiked with my guitar on my back across Ireland with a woman named Roisin, whom I met at a bus stop. We drank in pubs, where I led rousing sing-a-longs of "Me and Bobby McGee." Pubgoers chimed in during its memorable refrain about freedom being another word for nothing left to lose. The trip turned into an intense two-day love affair, unrequited but eye opening and life altering with lessons learned about women, adventure, and escapism. The tryst ended when we thumbed a ride with a truck driver. Roisin climbed into the cab, but before I did, the driver pulled away, leaving me standing there on the shoulder of the road, holding my guitar, waving goodbye to this woman whom I'd already convinced myself I loved. That episode taught me to view the world and my life as a big adventure story.

But now I see more humor in this story, and in all adventure stories, which I still love. As Joan Didion wrote, "We tell ourselves stories in order to live." I humbly offer this addendum to Didion's famous words: We tell stories to make sense of our lives. And, eventually, all stories about ourselves eventually stop working. We outgrow them. And, sometimes, when an old story we tell about ourselves fails us, when we no longer see ourselves in that story, we can find ourselves lost and in need of a new story. Unless we can scramble to come up with something fast, we can find ourselves adrift and unrecognizable to ourselves. God help us if this happens, because without an effective story as our guide, we are as good as dead. I know. Writing a new story can be the hardest thing to do—and yet sometimes we have no choice. Sometimes, our life depends on it.

It was October 1993 when I decided what I wanted to do next in my life. On a crisp Saturday morning, Di and I sat at a cafe, reading the *New York Times* and drinking coffee, when I announced my bold intentions.

"I think I'll work as an editor until I become a senior editor. Then, I want to do what our writers do. I want to be an adventure writer."

Di, a gifted editor and writer herself, looked up from her coffee and nodded yes. I felt her faith in me. And her faith in me reinforced something inside me. Faith in myself.

After that fateful morning conversation, I buckled down even harder at work. I knew I had the raw talent to become a successful adventure writer. I just needed a few more years of seasoning that I'd get from working as an editor. I'd already written a few feature stories, and I was developing my own writer's voice and even a theory about what MY version of an adventure story looked like. I loved kvetching and talking bullshit with complete strangers. People fascinated me, and I had a talent for putting them at ease. I had a vivid imagination, and I could turn anybody with a pulse into an amusing character. I also had an underlying theory that all stories were, at their root, love stories. We are all trying to feel seen, important, and loved—physically, emotionally, and spiritually. And though I wasn't afraid to throw an elbow at hypocrites or narcissists, I figured out how to tell an adventure story that celebrated the weird, the wonderful, and the very unusual. I was the Everyman, bumbling my way across the wild and making friends while doing it. I'd forget my raincoat and describe the plastic bag that I wore to keep dry. I was silly. I was fun. I was friendly.

Later that night, I fell asleep in bed with Di, thinking about all my past and future adventures. I remembered meeting Jon and our other top writers during a boat ride during the magazine's fifteenth anniversary party. That weekend, I tried to engage them in shoptalk. I also thought about the other established adventure writers I'd spoken to during my three years thus far working at *Outside*. I felt a kinship with them. Many of them seemed like paragons of tough, strong men. When I saw their pictures in the magazine, some of them seemed dapper and pulled together. Others appeared wild, unhinged even, with long, stringy hair, matted beard, and wild eyes that seemed to signal that they were deeply alive. That was me, or who I wanted to be, who I believed I already was, underneath my practiced, people-pleasing veneer. I wondered if they had difficult relationships with their fathers, too. I felt like all of us were bros.

Was it okay that I wasn't as tough and clear minded as them? Could I be successful as an adventure writer using humility, self-deprecation, and a winning smile? I knew I wasn't the next tough mountain climber. I would have to be the one and only Brad Wetzler.

During the winter of 1993–1994, I wrote the aforementioned pitch and shared it in a staff meeting. Everest had come up often in our editorial meetings. Of course it did. Sending writers to exotic, far-flung places and publishing their stories about their adventures is what we did. So, my story pitch didn't come forth from a vacuum. Everest was part of our office's zeitgeist. And yet it always had seemed off-limits, too extravagant, even to us. Extravagant—and also passé at the same time. Sure, it was the world's tallest mountain, but it wasn't the most difficult to climb by a long shot. We couldn't see how sending a writer to climb Everest would add anything new to the world of journalism.

Still, I was on fire for Everest. For the past couple years, I'd been monitoring Everest closely as my self-appointed job as head of *Outside's* adventure beat and as the assistant to the editor of the Dispatches section. I had been talking with sources who told me that Everest base camp had become a shit show. I had edited short articles about the growing numbers of climbers who were winding up on the summit on the same day. I am a deeply intuitive person. In my story pitch, I proposed sending a writer to the base camp on the "classic" southern Nepalese side. I mentioned Krakauer and climber and adventure journalist Greg Child. He was already an established Himalayan mountaineer. He seemed to me to be the logical choice for this truly extravagant story. My colleagues seemed enthusiastic about the idea. The timing seemed right, too. And then we editors got busy with other things, including our impending move to Santa Fe.

Me? I never forgot about the Everest base camp idea, and I planned to bug Mark about it as soon as we got settled in our new desert home.

five

A DIVINE PLAN

SOME THINGS IN LIFE HAPPEN FAST, WHILE OTHER THINGS TAKE time. I now understand that we don't have as much control as we like to think. The universe unfolds at its pace, and free will—if we have it—works in congruence with the pacing of the universe. I get why people talk about a divine plan. Some things require a person and the cosmos lining up. In the case of the Everest story, the universe turned out to be on its own schedule, and I simply followed along. As Di and I built a new life at the foot of the Sangre de Cristo Mountains, I occasionally found myself thinking about Everest. I needed to get moving on more feature assignments if I ever wanted to become a senior editor.

That spring, I traveled to LA for my first feature writing assignment. *Outside* didn't normally cover "hook and bullet" sports unless the scene was perfect. A senior editor named Alex Heard showed me a clip about bass fishermen going after record largemouths in a California reservoir; I made some calls and found a cast of characters. My Ahab was a young guy from Alabama who'd moved with his wife to California to catch the record fish. I had a white whale in the presumed-to-be-down-there big bass. And I had a villain, a hardass ex-cop. I flew to LA and spent four days fishing, and then wrote a story with the bodacious title "Big Bass and the Men Who Love Them." It was wildly popular. I did have a knack for writing features.

For a youngster on the staff, I had immense faith in my abilities. I'd already reported and written two features, and I'd already earned a bit of a reputation for my own spin on the adventure story. I didn't climb big peaks or go open-ocean sailing. I didn't need to. My go-to approach involved barely making any plans and showing up in a strange place surrounded by strange people and seeing what happened. And over several years, I developed serious chops in traveling alone and surviving in sketchy places. After the bass fishing story, I traversed chunks of the Appalachian Trail and exposed the exhausting, hilarious, and seemingly transformative lifestyle of being an AT thru-hiker. Another story, about the three weeks I camped in the woods drinking beer with Czech hobos, would be selected by Paul Theroux as one of the best adventure stories of 2001.

IN MAY 1994 OUTSIDE MOVED ITS HEADQUARTERS TO SANTA FE, NEW Mexico. Larry Burke, the magazine's owner and publisher, had bought a horse ranch outside town, and he was building a beautiful, stylish office building for the magazine in the Santa Fe Railyard. I'd visited Santa Fe once on a short vacation: the high-desert town seemed funky, artsy, and cool. As Di and I settled into living in a round split-level guesthouse on a ranch twenty-five minutes south of town, I was still thinking about the Everest base camp story, even as we were getting used to our new, more active lifestyle at the foot of the Sangre de Christo Mountains. I loved the vast, piñon-spotted landscape and the continuously clear big blue sky. We traded hot dogs and baseball for skis and mountain bikes, and we were happy to never spend another frigid winter in the Windy City.

During the next ten months, Mark and Jon talked occasionally about a possible Everest story, and Mark also began discussing financial details with Larry Burke. Meanwhile, I'd been researching commercial expeditions on both the northern Tibet side and the southern Nepal side, and copying Mark on my research. One windy, gray morning in March

1995, I stepped into Mark's office and poked him about the story. He usually had his head in a manuscript, and his first glance up betrayed the look of annoyance that all editors flash when pulled out of a story by a younger editor's questions. But then he smiled. "Let's do this. Call Jon and see if he's interested."

I hustled back to my office.

Here's how Krakauer tells the story in "Into Thin Air":

In March 1995 I received a phone call from an editor at *Outside* magazine proposing that I join a guided Everest expedition scheduled to depart five days hence and write an article about the mushrooming commercialization of the mountain and the attendant controversies. The magazine's intent was not that I climb the peak; the editors simply wanted me to remain in Base Camp and report the story from the East Rongbuk Glacier, at the foot of the Tibetan side of the mountain.

We talked for just a few minutes.

"You can write the story and never set foot in the Death Zone. What do you think?"

Krakauer seemed warm to the idea, and, before we ended the call, he said he'd consider the assignment, which excited me.

I was twenty-nine and, because of the hiking and sports I did, was more fit than I'd been during those frigid Chicago winters, but I was never a hardcore athlete. A dilettante, I was interested in other things besides sports and fitness: music, literature, yoga, even hanging out talking to artists and scientists in Santa Fe's many cafes.

I drove home, listening to Nirvana's *Nevermind*, to the small faux-adobe home that my now-wife Di and I bought for $140,000. I was elated.

I was bowled over by Cuba and Cosmo, our two rambunctious rescue puppies. Di and I hugged and headed across the road for a celebratory hike in the foothills. Dogs chasing rabbits, I filled Di in on the latest. A talented book editor working now at a small publishing company located across the Railyard within sight of my office, Di was thrilled by my news and told me about her new project editing a book by travel maven Rick Steves. We planned a weekend trip to White Sands and Carlsbad Caverns. We were young, happy, and in love. We were building a life together, and it was good. Life was *great*.

Krakauer did consider the story idea, and he even went so far as to book a flight and get the required immunizations.

I'm not sure how much time passed, but one afternoon Mark came into my office and told me that Krakauer had decided against the base camp story but was now considering going to Everest the following spring—and he wanted to climb to the top from the southern Nepalese base camp. This route was the more classic route that Sir Edmund Hillary had climbed in 1953.

Now I was thrilled. This wasn't the story I'd pitched back in 1994. It was a far more adventurous story. As exciting as the prospect of having an *Outside* writer on Everest seemed, I could tell that Mark was uncomfortable with the increased level of danger of the story. He feared losing his friend. And he reminded us of this. Winter set in, and the piñon-specked foothills glistened white under the bluebird sky. Di and I took our cross-country skis out of the closet and, our dogs in tow, glided around the mountain trails.

Mark gave me the assignment of calling various commercial guiding companies and trying to land him on one of them. In January 1996, in congruence with Mark, I got Krakauer confirmed with a Seattle-based outfit called Mountain Madness, led by the experienced mountaineer Scott Fischer, in exchange for a combination of cash and advertising space in *Outside*. And then, in late February, Rob Hall, of New Zealand–based Adventure Consultants, called me with a better offer. Mark called Jon and told him. The countdown to the spring 1996 Everest season began. I called Krakauer to wish him luck and asked him to stay safe.

During this period, I felt wildly alive. I was now thirty and an associate editor. These early, minimal conversations with Krakauer and Mark about this new story assignment made me feel like I was part of something big and exciting. And it *was* thrilling and fun. But I wasn't really doing anything except talking on the phone. Krakauer was the only guy with skin in this game: his life. And I knew that Mark was steering the ship of this new, bolder article.

I now see that I might have already gotten carried away. Those words "ego" and "grandiosity" again. I felt certain that once the Everest story hit the newsstands, I'd be promoted to senior editor. Once I secured that title, I could leave the magazine staff and hang my own shingle as an adventure writer. I planned to negotiate a contract to write three or four feature stories a year and then fill the rest of my schedule with stories at *GQ*, *Wired*, *National Geographic Adventure*, *Men's Journal*, and, with luck, the *New York Times*.

I felt ready to take on the world. Empowered. In retrospect, I was puffed up on hubris.

six

A PERFECT STORM

A S APRIL PROGRESSED, WE STOPPED HEARING FROM OUR
writer as he began the trek into base camp. With communications
limited, we followed Himalayan weather reports on the internet, and
Mark received updates from his wife, Linda Moore, who heard from him
via satellite phone once a week. Eventually, word came from Linda that
Krakauer and his team would make their summit bid on May 10.

As they made their way toward the summit, I certainly felt excited
but also scared. No, terrified. Of what? One of my tasks as the editor
who oversaw the adventure beat at *Outside* was writing obituaries of the
extreme athletes who pushed the limits too far. Would I end up writing an obituary about the writer *Outside* had sent to Mount Everest?
Was I freaking out on that May 1996 morning? Fuck yeah. We all were.
We paced the halls and swigged coffee. We chatted with friends on the
phone and made pointless trips to the Borders bookstore next door and
flipped through magazines. We did everything we could to distract ourselves. And when all the distracting failed to distract us? We fretted.

I tried to calm myself by breathing deeply. I worried. I might have
even prayed for his safety.

On the morning of May 10, 1996, the editors met in the hallway
for our daily morning meeting, where the managing editor buttonholed
us about deadlines. Mark, looking simultaneously frazzled and about to
burst with good news, cleared his throat.

"I heard from Linda last night. I have good news. Jon summitted just after noon, Everest time. Linda said he sounded good, strong. He's headed back now. As we all know, the most important, dangerous part of the climb is getting down."

High fives all around. I felt as happy and satisfied as I'd ever felt.

Looking back, I had little reason to be so happy. I didn't know it then, but as I sauntered back to my office slapping more high fives to the secretaries and receptionist, people I did not yet know but would soon learn about were dying.

I slept soundly that night. The next morning, Di and I were at a moving sale for Alex Heard, an editor who was leaving for New York to take a job at the *Times*. Alex came running out of the house, looking panicked.

"There's been an accident on Everest. Scott Fischer is dead. No word on Krakauer."

I nearly collapsed on the ground. Di and I jumped into my pickup and drove across town to the office. I landed in my chair and picked up the phone. I tried calling Adventure Consultants in New Zealand. I tried calling Mountain Madness, their competitor. I tried calling the editors of various mountain blogs as well as the *New York Times*. I didn't get anybody. Di went home, and a few of us worked the phones all day. No news. And then at around 3 p.m., Mark entered my office and told me that he'd heard from a source that Jon was still alive, though he had no further details.

At home I told Di the news. We held each other, and then we drove to Alex's going-away barbecue at the home of our colleague Hampton Sides and his journalist wife, Ann Goodwin Sides. Nobody was in the frame of mind for a party.

We stood in the quiet dark and nursed our beers, staring at the Milky Way, which in New Mexico looks like somebody spilled a pitcher of cream across the night sky. We were ten thousand miles from Everest, but it was as if we were at base camp too. We knew many of the people up there. I'd spoken to Fischer several times, on the phone and in person. As an editor, it's so easy to think of people as characters. Too easy. But that night, it became painfully obvious that they were flesh and blood, mortal and vulnerable. And they were dying. And our writer? He was huddled in a tent, maybe dying, too.

We sulked and moped and drank some more. And then Hampton's voice pierced the night sky.

"Mark. You have a phone call."

Looking stunned, Mark jogged inside. We waited in silence until he returned. "Um, Jon is okay. But Rob, his team leader, isn't. He stopped to stay with a sick client, and he's stuck there now. They may not make it through the night."

I'd spoken to Rob frequently that spring. He seemed so brave, friendly, and optimistic about the climb and about the future of guiding clients on Everest. And now, as I sat holding a plastic cup full of beer, he was dying of exposure on the South Summit, a place I had never visited but felt as if I knew. My mind raced. I knew the idea of rescue at night in a storm was beyond fantastical. But I still held out a glimmer of hope that somebody could do something. There's that psychological defense called denial again. No, nothing could save him. Rob was just below the summit of the world's tallest mountain. He might as well have been on the dark side of the moon. As my tired brain tried to grasp the grim reality, I felt as empty as a capsized sailboat whose adventurous solo captain was thrown overboard by a big wave off Antarctica. Our guy was safe in his tent, but he was still in the Death Zone, and he was nowhere near out of trouble. And I still felt sick.

The next morning, I talked to Mark. Rob Hall had died during the night. He and Fischer weren't the only fatalities. Over the next few days, we learned of the deaths of six other climbers. Other guides and clients were injured and badly frostbitten. Our writer was still alive and on his way back down the mountain. The weather looked clear for the next two days it would likely take him to descend. But as we were learning, on Everest, the situation can go south in a hurry.

Sad, rattled, but breathing a little easier knowing that our writer was likely out of the woods, we resumed our work of putting out a summer issue.

He arrived safely in base camp, and then I got his call from the hotel in Kathmandu. After I hung up the phone, I went for a walk. I took my first full deep breath in weeks. And then I took another.

In mid-August, *Outside* published "Into Thin Air," a seventeen-thousand-word account of the tragedy of the 1996 climbing season on Mount Everest. An ABC News team interviewed me in my office, and I spoke to scores of reporters for other news outlets, per Mark's request. And then, as I had planned, I gave notice, packed my things, and, in mid-December 1996, seven months after that intense month of May when we editors lived on the edge of our seats, I drove away from the *Outside* office and stepped into the rest of my life. My life appeared to be on the upswing. Man, is it easy to deceive ourselves.

seven

SWINGING THE WORLD
BY ITS TAIL

T HE LIFE OF A FREELANCE ADVENTURE WRITER WAS ALL I dreamed it would be. On the first Monday after New Year's Day 1997, I woke early and settled into my new home office: the spare bedroom of our small, starter home in Eldorado, a friendly, affordable subdivision outside Santa Fe. Sipping coffee, I sat on the edge of my seat, scrolling the pixelated headlines and stories on online news sites, scanning for mentions of people, places, and trends I might research and develop into a story. I looked out my window across the high desert, dotted with piñon pines, toward the Sandia and Jemez mountain ranges. I lost myself in the rusty dirt, the big blue sky, the broad views. All this natural beauty gave me a warm feeling in my belly. I thought about all the new and interesting friends I'd made: artists, writers, and misfits of various types. *I've arrived*, I thought. *Finally*. The future seemed bright. Di and I were in love, and we were stepping into our adult life together. After seven years of hard work at Northwestern's Medill School of Journalism and *Outside*, I had made it: I was an adventure writer.

I closed the browser and began drafting an email to Lonnie Dupre, a polar explorer from Minnesota, to let him know *Outside* had given me the green light to write a feature about him.

Dupre was planning to circumnavigate Greenland, the world's largest island, by kayak in the south and by dogsled in the frozen north. I had pitched the story as a study of the weird state of exploration in contemporary times. My driving question: *What's the point of an expensive, dangerous trip like this when almost everything has been achieved and mapped?* I saw Lonnie's corporate-backed expedition as both grandiose and a little pointless. The story's working title: "The End of Exploration."

"I have my plane ticket to Ottawa, and I'll meet you there in May," I wrote, finishing with, "Can't wait to join you in Greenland!"

I closed my email and opened a file containing the galleys of an article I'd written for *George* about a group of runners from the Indigenous Tarahumara people of Mexico's Sierra Nevada. I proofed the pages and emailed my editor Ned that I loved his tweaks and that the story was ready to print. Then I ended the morning with a phone call to Alex Heard, who was editing the front-of-the-book at the *New York Times*.

"What are you looking for these days?" I asked. "Are there any topics you want me to explore?" We chatted briefly, and I set down the phone. I felt accomplished, proud, and engaged, with a morning's work under my belt. What a dream.

As I opened the sliding glass door to the backyard, Cuba and Cosmo came trotting toward me. Together, we exited the gate and walked down a narrow trail across our sloped backyard into the arroyo behind our house. Cuba, a sleek, tan collie mix, sped ahead of us, leaping in the air, trying to spot rabbits over sagebrush and chamisa bushes. Cosmo, a stocky, loyal cattle dog / pit bull mix, stayed close to me, almost hugging my legs. But my mind was on Greenland and beyond. *What will it be like to stand on the Icecap? What will almost twenty-four hours of daylight be like? What will it be like to be free from full-time desk jockeying and live part of the year on the road?*

The dogs and I crossed the road and began hiking up a rocky trail in the forest preserve, headed to the top of the tallest foothills. As the dogs played, I sat on a rock and looked down at my little house and the vast high desert of northern New Mexico. Feelings of warmth and connection grew inside me, and at first they felt unfamiliar, even uncomfortable. I hoped they'd stick around a while. *Was it possible that life as a husband and homeowner would help me feel more solid and stable? Would life as a world-traveling adventure writer bring me the inner peace that had seemed so elusive to me as a kid and in my twenties? Or, at least, could this new life help me keep the chaos that filled my core and whispered its disruptive thoughts to me at bay?*

I headed down the mountain and back into my home office with Greenland still on my mind and a fragile confidence about succeeding in this new world. My anxieties and concerns felt like little secrets I could get away with having. If I didn't mention them, they wouldn't exist.

I kept my head down. I continued pursuing my work. And I leaned on hope that the periods of depression that had afflicted me since my teen years would stop recurring—or that the pills my doctor prescribed to treat them would actually, finally manage them well enough that I could live out my dream.

The weeks and months passed by, and I wrote one solid adventure story after the next. By the end of Year 1, I'd spent three weeks in Greenland on assignment for *Outside* and three weeks reporting on Russia's secretive space program at Star City outside Moscow for *George,* and I'd traveled extensively across the United States for various other magazines. I'd partied with cosmonauts in Moscow's discos, dug for dinosaur bones with Republican congressperson Newt Gingrich in Montana, investigated Bill and Hillary Clinton's tight friendships with a lawyer for Tyson Foods in Arkansas. I'd traveled inside Colorado's Cheyenne Mountain, home of the highly secretive US missile defense system. I'd stood in a major league locker room interviewing Cy Young Award–winning pitcher Greg Maddux. I'd interviewed NBA players and several Olympians. I capped off the year by sitting for a live interview with an MSNBC newscaster about my *George* magazine article about high-stakes drama on the Mir space station. In my first thrilling year as a freelance writer, I spent four months on the road and published feature articles in GQ, Men's Journal, Outside, George, and a couple of shorter pieces in the New York Times.

Fall turned to winter. Di and I enjoyed our first Christmas together without traveling to see family. We hiked with the dogs. We ate enchiladas at Santa Fe's renowned restaurants. We enjoyed nights out with friends at saloons. On January 2, 1998, I was back at my desk in my home office, scanning the high desert, the distant mountains, and my own inner landscape. I felt a deep sense of satisfaction. I'd done it. I'd pulled it off. I'd become a world-traveling adventure writer who was also dipping into political writing as well. And all of this had happened in only a year. If Year 1 was this successful, then what would Year 2 bring? What would Years 5 and 10 bring? The prospect felt intoxicating. I was doing this! What next? A book? Maybe a film deal? My older writer friends were already finding this type of massive success. They were landing $500,000 book deals, $500,000 movie deals. Why not me?

I looked up at my email inbox and noticed a message from Ned, my editor at George: "Call me."

I heard Ned's smart, warm voice. "Hey, Brad. I was talking with John"—John F. Kennedy Jr., the magazine's cofounder, publisher, and editor in chief—"We want to make you a contributing editor. What do you think?"

"Hell, yeah!" I said.

This was fabulous news. I was already a correspondent at Outside; a contributing editor title at George was yet more confirmation that I was doing great work and that I was on a solid path to the future I envisioned for myself.

"We want your first article to be a profile of Senator Paul Wellstone, of Minnesota."

We said goodbye and hung up. A few days later, I received a contract to write several stories in the coming year, and in return I'd be paid $100,000. I also received a handwritten note in the mail from Kennedy. It read:

Dear Brad, I just wanted to write and informally welcome you as a contributor to the magazine. We're very pleased to have you aboard, and we hope you have as much fun putting it together as we do. Good luck on Sen. Wellstone—the photos are great. Best, John Kennedy

This sure felt like success. So what if I was starting to navigate some major inner turmoil? On the outside, everything was looking up.

eight

TREMORS

O N A SUNNY AND COOL MID-JANUARY DAY IN 1998, I DROVE AN hour north of Santa Fe to the town of Villanueva. I pulled off the highway near a favorite fly-fishing spot, donned my rubber waders, and, with rod in hand, waded out into the cold, knee-high water. I took a wet fly from my khaki vest and threaded the fine nylon leader through the eye. Or, rather, I tried to. I missed my first attempt. I held the fly closer to my eyes and tried a second time. I missed again. I tried again. And again. I spent the next five minutes trying to push the leader through the tiny eye, to no avail.

I walked back out of the river and sat down on the rocky bank. I held my breath to quiet my body, arms, and hands, and tried again. *Yes!* I did it. I waded into the river once more, cast toward a small, V-shaped rapid near the opposite bank, and watched the fly float downstream. When my line straightened out, I pulled my arm back. Fly and line lifted from the water and looped behind me. I moved my arm forward and the line soared back out toward the same watery V. I felt a tug and jerked up, hoping to feel the heft of a trout. But instead I'd hooked a small branch. Ordinarily, snagging a branch is no big deal; it's part of fly fishing. But I was already frustrated from spending nearly fifteen minutes tying on the fly. I waded out to the branch, took out my pocketknife, and cut the leader. There were other flies and more leader in my vest, but I'd had it. I wasn't up for another fifteen minutes of frustration.

I turned toward the bank and left the river, took off my waders, and set my fly rod in the back of my truck. I saw a coyote on the bank plunge its head into a hole and pull out a large, gray jackrabbit by the neck. It gave its catch a single, fatal shake and disappeared behind a chamisa bush into an arroyo. I started my truck and headed back toward the house.

Back at home, I made a cup of tea and lay down on the couch. I turned on a college football game that I couldn't care less about and petted Cosmo, feeling sorry for myself. Di, dressed in jeans and a Michigan sweatshirt, came in from the garden. She came over and asked what was wrong.

"I couldn't even tie the fly onto my leader."

"Because of the tremor?"

"Yeah. It's gotten worse in the past months."

"I know. I've noticed. I didn't say anything."

"I've noticed it, too."

A hand tremor is a common side effect of lithium. I'd been taking 300 milligrams of the mood stabilizer every day for nine years. It wasn't the only drug I took regularly. I also took 120 milligrams of Prozac — 40 milligrams more than the recommended maximum dose; 450 milligrams of Wellbutrin, another antidepressant, the maximum recommended; Dexedrine, a stimulant, to treat the sedating side effects of the other drugs; fluvoxamine, for the looping, obsessive, self-critical thoughts I complained about; lorazepam, for anxiety; propanolol, a beta blocker, which reduces physical symptoms of anxiety; and trazodone, an antidepressant with sedating side effects, for insomnia.

———

MY FIRST VISIT to a mental health professional took place in 1989 in Prairie Village, Kansas, the suburb of Kansas City where I grew up. Dennis, a close friend of my parents, made the appointment for me. A high-powered businessperson who suffered from mild to moderate depression, he'd sought the advice of a psychiatrist named Dr. Jerry, who diagnosed him with bipolar disorder after a couple of visits and prescribed medications. Dennis would later reject the diagnosis, but not before he encouraged me to see Dr. Jerry, too, after my mother shared with him a bit about my struggles with depression. She must have told him about my father's heavy drinking, too, because Dennis, who at the time was attempting to come to terms with his own childhood in an alcohol-infused dysfunctional family, invited me to join him at several Adult Children of Alcoholics meetings that summer.

I drove myself to Dr. Jerry's office and sat down in a white leather chair. The office, with its wood paneling, soft leather furniture, and shelves full of books, felt homey to me. Dr. Jerry was nerdy but hip. He looked a little like Art Garfunkel. I was impressed and flattered that he seemed to pay close attention to me and my stories. After only five minutes or so, I began sharing intimate details about my life, things I'd never told anyone before. And it felt really good, freeing, as if I were unloading bags of rocks from some inner backpack of my psyche. He asked pointed questions about my moods. I told him how lonely and depressed I felt at home. He didn't ask me about my parents, and I didn't volunteer any information about my father's drinking. I also didn't tell him that my mother frequently updated me about my father's long-term, on-again, off-again affair. Both my parents had instructed me not to say a word to "anybody, not a soul," and I felt obligated to keep those secrets. More than that, I felt confused and scared about what the consequences might be should I let the family secrets slip out. My parents knew a lot of important people in town. I was too scared to even tell my best friend. And so, I talked—no, I blabbed—freely about my own life. How I drove my VW bus out to a friend's farm and camped alone there instead of going to college parties. Dr. Jerry scribbled in his notebook.

"Do you ever feel *too* good?" he asked.

"Too good? What do you mean by that?" I was confused; wasn't the problem here that I didn't feel good?

"Do you feel so good that you do risky things that endanger you or other people? Risky sex? Risky stunts? Spend money you don't have?"

"Ha, well, I'm a twenty-three-year-old college student. I don't have any money."

"Think about it."

I did.

"Well, I once attended a nudist party at college. I took mushrooms once, too. When I was a teenager, I sometimes felt so close to God that I felt as if I was merging with him."

He scribbled harder.

"Sometimes I go on long drives in my bus, and I feel a sense of freedom. Ecstasy even. It feels so good to be on the road and free of my family's bullshit."

He scribbled more.

I'm sure a few other things were said, but I don't remember. Then, as my fifty minutes was about to expire, Dr. Jerry set down his notebook.

"Brad," he said, "you have bipolar disorder."

"Okay," I said. I felt confused but also glad that my problems apparently had a name.

Dr. Jerry spent five minutes telling me that bipolar disorder was a sickness of my brain. "You have a chemical imbalance, and that's what's causing your wild mood swings," he said.

I was compliant. "Okay."

Dr. Jerry stood up and handed me a white slip of paper.

"What's this?"

"It's a prescription for lithium, Brad. You can fill this at any Walgreens. It's inexpensive and will stop the extreme mood swings."

Extreme mood swings? He'd said those words twice. And though I said "okay," his description of my mind and life didn't resonate as truth for me. Or did it? I did lose my temper with my family sometimes. My mom and dad said that I'd really changed since the days when I was a bright, happy little kid. But wait—hadn't I been unhappy at home for good reasons? Like, because my dad drank until he passed out and couldn't be woken up? And my mom would come to me crying, asking for hugs and advice about leaving my dad? And what about the lies? I had figured out through a little sleuthing that my dad had a spare apartment for his girlfriend. When I shared this with my mother, she ransacked it. And then told me not to tell a soul about any of it. Mood swings? The doctor's words stung badly.

As confused as I was, I said nothing. This label was for someone else, yet I took the prescription from Dr. Jerry's hand and stuck it in my pants pocket. Thanking him, I walked out of his office to my bus. I felt scared—but weirdly hopeful. *Maybe this is what's been going on with me all these years*, I thought. Maybe my family isn't really that bad, and maybe I'm not that bad. Maybe I just have some faulty chemistry in my brain, and, as Dr. Jerry said, this drug will fix it. I drove straight to Walgreens and filled the prescription. That night, I stood in front of the bathroom mirror, removed the bottle's white cap, poured out a single pink lithium pill, and popped it into my mouth. As I swallowed the pill, I felt a surge of excitement. *I've just swallowed the end to my depression!* No more feeling unhinged and angry. Suddenly, the future seemed bright.

I didn't notice much except that I felt a little numb. I took another pill at noon the next day and another at bedtime.

Three months later, I moved to Chicago to start graduate studies. Dr. Jerry kept refill prescriptions coming, but after six months he called to tell me that he was retiring and I'd need to find a new psychiatrist. My insurance company picked one for me: Dr. Walt, an earnest, chubby, fresh-faced resident in psychiatry at Northwestern's medical school, who a few months earlier had burned a wart off my hand as my primary care doctor.

At our first meeting, Dr. Walt smiled as I told him about my diagnosis of bipolar and my new life at Northwestern. He nodded his head as if to show empathy and agreement. At the end of our first session, he told me he'd continue writing me lithium prescriptions. (I've since learned the term "diagnostic momentum." Doctors tend to take the previous diagnoses made by other doctors at face value.) He also said he thought I'd benefit from taking another drug, new on the market. "It's called Prozac," he said. "It seems as if depression is your bigger issue. It should help."

I took the medications religiously, despite their overall ineffectiveness. They didn't stop the swirling emotions. They didn't help me better navigate personal and business relationships, which continued to be scary and difficult. I didn't know how to do them. I rushed in. I pulled away. I blamed the other person. They would leave. And then I would be alone. Utterly alone. And then? I blamed myself. I scolded myself. I cursed myself. And sometimes I became so depressed I couldn't move.

Throughout college, I suffered extreme bouts of depression that left me immobilized on the couch for weeks. One led me to withdraw from college during my sophomore year. I couldn't get up to get to class. My three roommates went about their lives: studying, cooking meals, dating, having parties around me on the couch. Eventually, I found enough inspiration to walk down to campus and sign the withdrawal papers. It took all the energy I had.

But throughout these experiences, I stayed devoted to, practically in love with, psychiatry. The various doctors I met with, all of them seemingly empathic, progressive men, listened intently about my inner and outer experiences. My father had rarely listened to me, at least not about the things that mattered to me or how I felt, and I didn't confide much in my friends. These sessions always felt like a release. Each meeting ended with the same ritual: I signed a check; the doctor signed a prescription. They got what they wanted, and I got what I wanted: empathy and something that felt as close to fatherly love as I'd ever felt.

I loved psychiatry, and it's safe to say psychiatry loved me. I had faith in the idea that pills were the answer to my problems. As a journalist, I trusted scientific answers, and I trusted men in white coats who expressed empathy and concern with furrowed brows, men who nodded their heads when I talked about my life. That kind of reaction to my thoughts and expressed feelings was new to me. The positive attention felt nothing less than fantastic.

And so began an adventure story that would run parallel to the story of how I became an adventure writer. Perhaps you could call it *Adven-*

tures in Psychiatry: How I Sold My Soul to the Medical Establishment.
But whatever the title, I had to live it. And it almost killed me.

————

THE TREMOR WAS undeniable. I was glad that my editors and colleagues weren't seeing me much in person. Yes, let's talk about denial. I read an article in a psychology journal recently suggesting that we humans are only 5 percent conscious. This means that 95 percent of our thinking selves, including our memories, remains unconscious, buried within us somewhere, silenced and festering. If true, this fact is mind blowing. And it would explain why, as Year 2 of my adventure-writing career unfolded, I was able to reflect so positively on Year 1, when, in fact, it had been hard.

Depression is the number one reason people seek help from therapists and psychiatrists, yet it remains a puzzle to doctors and drug manufacturers. There are countless theories about its causes and a billion-dollar industry organized around its treatment with medications. But the truth is, nobody knows why or how most common antidepressants work, or why they don't work, or why they work for a while and then stop working. And the jury is out on how much they even help. Recent studies suggest that the efficacy of Prozac and similar drugs is less than 50 percent.

Yet prescription drugs remain the go-to treatment. As for the causes? Experts used to say it was faulty brain chemistry, perhaps due to genetics. But more and more studies show that a major cause of depression is toxic shame. And toxic shame is a common symptom of childhood trauma. The Adverse Childhood Experiences scale quantifies growing up with various forms of parental neglect as correlated to carrying toxic shame. Regular shame is a normal emotion. Whereas guilt is an uncomfortable, internal feeling of remorse about a specific act or behavior, shame says your whole self is unworthy and bad. Shame is self-disgust and feeds on your very identity. It becomes particularly devastating when the impact to your sense of self is ongoing. Toxic shame opens the door to the room where you always feel small and worthless. It can trickle into your inner dialogue, like a poison, locking you into a painful loop of negative self-talk. When this kind of shame lingers without resolution, the desire to hide from it or escape from yourself can lead to potentially harmful behaviors like substance misuse or self-harm.

Looking back on my journey today, I believe that toxic shame was the source, the core, of most of my problems. When a child is asked to hold family secrets—like my father's blackout drinking and his betrayals of my mother—a child will direct the blame for the family's dysfunction back onto himself. He will scapegoat *himself* to save the family. Why does this happen? A child cannot risk being disconnected from a parent. Given the choice between blaming a parent, who exists as a kind of god in a child's psyche, or blaming himself, the child will choose himself. To my mind, the canoeing incident was not the cause of my family's dysfunction, but it solidified and highlighted an experience in me that has been a constant thread. First, my father shut down any conversation about my near drowning and denied it had even happened. I was forced to process the violent episode myself, so I blamed myself. It was the same story with his drinking and romantic betrayal of my mother, about which my mother confided in me. No child should have to be brave enough to risk the consequences of such a confrontation: being pushed out of the family system. The more I tried to tell the truth, the more I was pushed out, blamed, and shamed.

Given no other options, I agreed to the blame. And that self-blame, that habitual, blaming voice, grew into a brutal, muscular, and ruthless inner critic.

And now, at age thirty-one in 1997, I was a likable man. I knew this. I was friendly, fun, energetic, and kind. But I hated myself. I didn't want to risk being close to anybody in case they judged me, which would make me hate myself even more than I already did. I liked having acquaintances, but I didn't know how to be a good friend. I didn't know how to pick a good friend. I made friends with misfits. I told myself, *We all have good souls. So why shouldn't I be friends with the deranged meth user on the corner? He might have some wisdom to offer, right?* He sure did, but I chose him over people who were solid and would be good to me, who would see me. I didn't think I deserved goodness, and I didn't want to be seen.

The adventurous travel-writing lifestyle didn't just afford me the persona my ego needed: it let me be anonymous. It protected me from intimacy. I didn't create a literal alter ego. I didn't lie about who I was on the road. But I reveled in chatting with strangers in bars and cafes. If I didn't know a person and there were no worries about maintaining a relationship in the future, I could let myself feel deeply connected, even intimate with them, even if I'd known them for only five minutes. And then I could walk away. I even came to believe that this was the purest form of intimacy—that temporary hit, that quick euphoric high. And while I didn't physically cheat on Di during my travels, I cheated emotionally on her every day I was on the road, joining up with women to explore the countryside or urban markets, turning on the charm, flirting, and enjoying the reciprocated attention.

I just *needed a lot of space*: this was my story line about my avoidance behavior. I wasn't very aware of the sensations in my body. If you talked to my family, they would say I was naive. I was disorganized and depressed. But I was able to cover it all up by leaning on my verbal and writing abilities. I showed up with a smile and told people I was doing great, and because I was expert at acting the part, they believed me. It was almost too easy, which made it even worse.

But I wasn't doing great.

Even on the road, even as my career was taking off and I was wrapping up a successful Year 2, I was getting lonelier and lonelier every day.

That river in Arkansas—the roaring sound in my ears, the feeling of the strong current pushing me into the submerged log, those minutes of simultaneous violence, panic, and weird calm—that psychic roar followed me everywhere. There's a line in *Siddhartha* that always gets me: "The river is everywhere." It certainly is.

The river inside me was post-traumatic stress disorder, PTSD, but I couldn't see that yet. I was still being swept along by it, pretending I was walking on solid ground.

nine

CRACKS IN THE ARMOR

M Y ARTICLE ABOUT LONNIE DUPRE'S GREENLAND EXPEDITION
became my first magazine cover story. It was published in September 1997 and included a picture of a gnarly adventurer hanging from a climbing rope. For all appearances, the piece was a success, and I was off to a great start as an adventure writer.

But the two stories I'm about to tell you I've never told anyone, not even my close friends:

In early May 1997, I flew to Ottawa, Canada, where I met Lonnie, John Holscher, and Lonnie's wife, Kelly. From Ottawa we flew to Iqaluit, Baffin Island, where we boarded another flight for Narsarsuaq, Greenland. As we crossed the Arctic Circle, Lonnie poured vodka into shot glasses and we toasted each other like explorers of yore. In Narsarsuaq we took yet another flight for Nuuk, where at last we passed out in our sleeping bags in a rock quarry near the airport. The next morning, we skipped southward in a helicopter, and then a second helicopter. We arrived in Paamiut three days after I left Santa Fe.

The very next morning, Lonnie told me that he and Holscher had decided to leave immediately rather than spending several days getting their gear in order, as they'd promised me they'd do months before. They boarded their kayaks and waved goodbye. I took pictures and videos as they paddled out of sight, then boarded an eighteen-foot Boston Whaler motorboat I'd hired to follow them. My guide and driver was a tall, muscular Inuit man wearing a Helly Hansen dry suit and Sorel boots. He steered the Whaler through long, lightning-shaped cracks in the ice. When the leads became too narrow for our boat, he'd pull out a metal pole, insert it between slabs of ice, and pry and push. The boat would tilt 30 degrees, 45 degrees. I'd clutch a thick braided rope to stay aboard. More than once, the Whaler became stuck. Again the driver would pry and push. I'd scramble to the starboard stern to shift our center of gravity, and then, grasping the coaming, I'd hurry back to the port stern. Occasionally the bow shot completely out of the water, and the entire front end landed with a thud on the ice. Other times, the stern shot skyward and landed with a thud on the ice. More than once, I became convinced we were stuck, fucked, and would need a rescue. But my driver never seemed to lose faith. He wouldn't stop prying and shifting his weight or barking orders at me to move my ass to the starboard or port. And, sure enough, we would become unstuck exactly as he'd expected. We'd get through the icy eye of whatever needle we happened to be trying to thread. We proceeded like this all day. And then we camped on a beach underneath soaring cliffs and surrounded by icebergs and pack ice. It felt so remote, so beautiful, that I was filled with both awe and terror: *mysterium tremendum et fascinans* — a mystery before which humans tremble in fascination, both repelled and attracted.

The next morning, we lit out again in pursuit of Lonnie and John. But by noon the driver and I agreed with a knowing look that we'd lost them. At the end of Day 2, we turned the Boston Whaler around and headed back toward Paamiut. Clearly, Lonnie and Holscher were making great progress. I'd only been gone a week, but my work was done.

It took two days to return to Paamiut. I thanked my guide and walked back to my campsite. There was a note on my tent that I couldn't stay there, so I packed up and hiked outside the town and set up camp on a beach under a high fjord. It was a picture-perfect place. The next morning, I hiked into town and stopped by the helicopter pad. Nobody was there, but there was a sign on the shack that served as the ticketing counter. I had gotten it into my head that the helicopters flew every week on Wednesdays. So, why did this sign say the next flight out was undetermined?

Undetermined? What does that mean? I felt a twinge of anxiety.

I tried calling a phone number, but the person who answered didn't speak English. I always preferred keeping things loose and flexible; I took some egotistical pride in just winging it, flying by the seat of my adventurous pants. Lonnie had told me that flights went out every week, and I believed him. I was moving too fast, climbing too quickly, to fact-check this essential point of how I was going to get out of this remote part of the world. Clearly, Lonnie didn't know either. I'd prepared in every way but this.

Back at my campsite, I rummaged through my backpack and found a package of freeze-dried beef stroganoff. I boiled water on my camp stove and mixed in the contents. The noodles and beef were salty but tasty. Cleanup involved scrubbing the grease out of the pots and pans with beach gravel and then again with soap. A piece of dark chocolate served as dessert. Throughout dinner and cleanup, I maintained calm. As the midnight sun hovered at 15 degrees over the western horizon, I gazed up at Mars and Venus, bright dots along the zodiac against the cyan sky. I breathed a sigh of relief that my inner Abyss hadn't raised its debilitating head. I felt proud, too. What a fucking amazing few days.

I grew sleepy. I crawled inside my tent and zipped my thin thirty-one-year-old body into my mummy bag so that only my face was exposed to the cold night air. I even nodded off. But as soon as I lost consciousness, I felt a jolt in my legs. I felt a lump in my throat. I felt my stomach clench. The Abyss. It was back.

The Abyss was a pitlike sensation in my solar plexus that felt like utter aloneness and left me feeling panicked for human connection. Over time, it could grow both in depth and intensity until I felt consumed. Roaring like the White River and simultaneously as silent as outer space, it led me to thrash for escape, but escape wasn't possible. I was probably thirteen or fourteen years old the first time I experienced the Abyss. I was sitting by my drunk father's side in the living room of our house. It visited me often during my travels and life. And when it wasn't present in full, I could feel the edge it. Looking back, I can see that my fear of its return drove much of my behavior, sometimes clinging to people and things. Other times, running from them.

I attempted to keep the Abyss at bay with deep breathing exercises. But the Abyss was alive in my body now. *Jesus Christ, calm down, Brad,* I scolded myself, but with the opposite effect. My body convulsed. The solidness of flesh, bone, organ drained out of my torso, and the empty dark feeling that was always present but that I had learned to keep at bay metastasized, first slowly and then rapidly. My body, every cell, emptied out until I was the Abyss. I felt the urgency to move. No, thrash. I tugged at my sleeping bag, trying to escape its mummy-like clutches. I yanked it off my legs. I grabbed the tent zipper with my fist and, tearing the stitching, yanked it down. Outside, I crouched on all fours, sweating, huffing and puffing. I didn't know it then—I wouldn't understand for two more decades—but I was in the grips of a full-blown PTSD episode. The past wasn't the past. The past was alive inside my body and mind. I was no longer in Greenland. I was stuck on the log in the middle of the White River, the current pressed my skinny torso into the immovable log while the river clawed at my spindly limbs to be free. The push. The pull. The Abyss. The roar of the current echoed in my ears. A sharp submerged branch gouged into my skin. My father stood alone on the beach, frozen. Why won't you come get me? Fuck, then if you aren't coming, go get help! I looked up at the blue sky and raged at God. Save me. And then, as if watching a highlight film on the screen of my mind, I was no longer in the river. I was sitting on the couch in my living room, trying to do my homework. I was fifteen or sixteen. My father sat in his La-Z-Boy in full recline. A tall tumbler full of gin rested on the table next to him. He hadn't spoken in two hours. His mouth was agape like that of a corpse at the moment of death before anybody has bothered to gently close it for public viewing. His thick tongue was hanging out. Was he alive or dead? When was Mom due home from Junior League?

Or did I forget that she'd already come home and avoided my father and me in the living room and gone straight to bed? Where was my brother? Where was my sister? Why was I here alone with him, night after night? Who was in charge here?

———

HERE'S THE SECOND story I've never told anyone:

Depression always arrived first as fatigue.

A year later, while on assignment for *George* to write the Paul Wellstone profile, I arrived late at my hotel in Georgetown and went to bed immediately. When my alarm sounded at 7 a.m., I hit snooze. And I hit snooze again ten minutes later. I felt so fatigued, so exhausted, I couldn't get out of bed. I felt as if I'd been hit by a bus. Eventually I opened my eyes and turned on the television, hoping the sound would help rouse me, and then stood in the shower, hoping the hot water would knock me back into my mind and body. I toweled off and got dressed lethargically, finally realizing what was going on. Yet again, I'd been fooled into thinking I was just tired and overworked. *Fuck*, I thought. *Here we go again.* I opened the bottles of various medications and took an extra Prozac and an extra Dexedrine, thinking that might solve the problem.

I called Di and told her how I felt. My words barely made sense to myself, and I struggled to make sense of her response. The fogginess in my head and the heaviness in my body made me feel this was going to be a particularly nasty depression. *How the fuck am I going to finish this assignment? I can't lie in bed all day. I've got to be sharp.*

I threw on a coat and tie and took a taxi to the Capitol. The rain had stopped, and I was an hour early. I was already craving a nap. If I could just rest for thirty minutes, I believed I'd rejuvenate. I spotted a patch of grass under a leafy tree on the north side of the building. I spread my jacket on the ground and lay on my back, staring up at the cloudy sky. I set the alarm on my watch for noon, thirty minutes from now—or I thought I did—and lay back. I must have fallen asleep before my head found the ground. The next thing I knew, raindrops were splattering my face. I opened my eyes and looked at my watch. One o'clock. I'd slept for an hour and was now thirty minutes late for my meeting. I stood up, threw on my coat, and jogged across the street. I took the elevator up, then burst into the office, my coat wrinkled, my eyes puffy.

"Hi, I'm Brad Wetzler. Here to see Senator Wellstone."

"We wondered what happened to you. The senator is at the Capitol Cafe, meet him there."

What I didn't say was, "I'm sorry, I am falling fast into a desperate depression, and I went to sleep in a park." What I didn't say was, "The mistakes are starting to get too big for me to bounce back from." What I didn't say was, "I'm scared. I take more pills every month. I don't think I am okay."

What I said was, "Thanks," and ran back across the street to the Capitol. I went through the motions of the interview. I concentrated as hard as I could. All I needed was a couple of scenes for my story. All I needed was to keep propping myself up long enough to continue my facade of being okay.

ten

THE DREAM CONTINUES
(SORT OF)

DESPITE THE CRACKS IN THE ARMOR, I CONTINUED TO PUSH toward my goals, which remained the same: publish more articles in major magazines and keep my eyes open for ideas I could turn into a book. I pitched and wrote adventure stories that were well received. Editors courted me to write pieces, including an op-ed in the *New York Times* and reviews for the *New York Times Book Review*. Agents in New York called to see whether I was sitting on any book ideas (I told them I didn't have any—yet). I turned down job opportunities at magazines.

I stayed clear with my ambition; I felt as if I was on the path that I'd chosen, or maybe that had chosen me. But I was fueled by envy, too. I watched as my friends continued to have success with books and then sell movie rights. They moved out of Eldorado and into bigger houses in the foothills. It wasn't the money or the houses that made me churn on the inside; it was their new status within the world of writers, editors, and publishers. I continued to pitch and write adventure stories and, increasingly, political stories for *George*, and continued to be driven by a longing to be known and admired as a writer. It felt like there was a hole that no amount of publication credits could fill.

This envy was expected of me culturally. We spend our twenties and thirties trying to become somebody—acquiring expertise, status, things. I was playing the game, too, and fortunately, at the time, there was money in the quirky niche of my line of work. The internet was here to stay, but it hadn't yet usurped the place of analog publishing. Print was still king; magazines still sold ads; and therefore, there were large budgets to pay us writers—even to travel. Of course, this would all change with the 2008 financial crisis, but we didn't know that yet. I was in that rare group who made a living as a writer, and for those of us who had the chops and the experience, it wasn't a pauper's life. At $10,000 a story, you could string together a decent living by writing eight or so stories a year.

In 1999, I landed a feature story for the *New York Times* that sent me to Hawaii to interview Gene Savoy, a self-described old-school explorer who rediscovered major archeological sites and abandoned cities in South America. Savoy was thought to be the inspiration for the Indiana Jones character—and he was more controversial. Unlike Indiana Jones, he wasn't an educated archeology professor; he was a renegade. He was accused of grave robbery, keeping his discoveries to himself, and selling precious archeological findings. He also held controversial theories about interactions among ancient cultures that went against conventional theories and agreed-upon histories. Finally, he was a cult leader. After his toddler son died in Peru—either in an avalanche or from cholera—Savoy proclaimed that the child had been the reincarnation of Jesus Christ. Back in the States, he started a religious sect called the International Community of Christ, in which his savior son was the key figure, and Savoy was the ordained bishop.

My visits with him were fascinating, strange, and often sad. He was a heavy drinker and a raconteur. He was an original. I spoke with him often with a coterie of beautiful blonde women in swimsuits. One story I never forgot.

He told me that while exploring in the cloud forests of Peru, he and his support team became lost in the jungle. Each day, they hacked their way with machetes further into the jungle in search of a lost, pre-Incan city; each day the jungle seemed to grow back, covering up their route back out to civilization. After weeks of this, they were disoriented. Utterly lost.

One morning, while Savoy was in his tent looking at maps, he heard a sound like a bell ring out, and, as he told it, his ears perked up. He ran out of his tent to find the source of the sound. One of his men raised his hand. Savoy grabbed his machete and hacked at the vegetation where the man had been working.

Riiing.

Savoy hacked harder. *Riiing. Riiing.*

Savoy stopped and cleared away vines with his hands. A shiny, gray stone appeared underneath. And then another. And another.

He ordered his team to continue clearing away the vegetation. By midday, out of the dense jungle, an ancient Incan road emerged.

As I sat listening to Savoy, I was still confused about where the story was going. *Okay,* I thought, *They found an ancient road, but they are still miles from civilization.*

Savoy must have seen the puzzled look on my face. He grabbed my hand and looked into my eyes.

"Mr. Bradley, a road. Don't you get it?"

"But it was still in the middle of nowhere."

"Mr. Bradley, a road goes someplace. The Incan roads are linked up with villages and even with modern roads and highways. I knew we were saved. If we followed it far enough, it would lead us out. As long as we were in the jungle hacking through, we existed in chaos. It was hopeless. But if we stayed on the road, we would be saved. A road goes someplace."

It would be a decade before I understood the significance of that quote. It would take falling into a drug-fueled coma. It would take sitting by the body of a friend who'd died by suicide and watching his body taken away in an orange bag. Savoy seemed like an alcoholic wreck of a man—and that part of him I didn't admire—but he had seen the world. He had lived on the edge and close to death. Eventually, the wisdom of his words would be revealed to me through the jungle of my life, as I launched my journey of self-exploration. It would keep me on my path of healing. It would keep me going to yoga classes and sitting on my meditation cushion. It would keep me committed to the process of healing in moments that I wanted to give up. *A road goes someplace.*

Later that year, I wrote a story about Capt. Craig Button, an air force pilot who peeled off from his squadron during a training run in Arizona and flew his plane to Colorado, where he crashed into a mountain in a suicide. In reporting the story, I tried to crawl inside the mystery pilot's mind. I traveled to Texas, New York, Arizona. Last, I rented a car and then a single-engine plane and pilot in Rifle, Colorado, and traced his unhinged flight path during which he dropped unarmed bombs on national forests. I tried so hard to merge with him that I lost sight of my job, which was merely to write a five-thousand-word investigative magazine piece. I think I felt like solving the mystery of his death would help me solve the mystery of my life and unhappiness. I kept sloppy, handscrawled notes everywhere: in the kitchen, in the glove box of my car, on the palm of my hand. On the date the article was due, I sent off a steaming heap of a story that made no sense to even me. I knew I was on thin ice with *George*. Surely, I'll bluff my way out of this conundrum and write an amazing second draft, I told myself.

As I was waiting to hear back from Ned, I got a call from Alex Heard, who by then was an editor at *Wired*, asking if I would travel to India to write about cultural adjustments accompanying the tech boom. This was 1999, and young Indians—and even women!—were landing good jobs. The influx of money was upsetting the apple cart of a very traditional, mostly agrarian society. Women were losing the incentive to marry young or to marry the men their parents chose for them. There was suddenly unprecedented access to big houses and fancy cars. Women who'd grown up in poverty were making enough to get breast implants. Of course, I wanted to write the story and get a clip in *Wired*, so I said yes right away.

I had longed to travel to India for a few years, but for very different reasons. My yoga practice at home had grown more serious. Four or five days a week, I was practicing at Santa Fe Community Yoga Center. At the front of the room, there was a table with pictures of Indian sages and saints. I was both drawn to and confused by the images on this altar. I was a journalist; my work was based on facts. I believed then, and still do, in science and its many benefits. Why was I so drawn to these saints? Why was I drawn to Gene Savoy and his wacky spiritual theories?

Now I can see that I've always had an appreciation for the nonlogical and the nonlinear—for some sort of mystical thread that was carrying me through. If science is pulling things apart into smaller pieces to understand them, I was on board with that. But that's not the only way to work with information about the world. Any scientist will tell you that the whole is different from the sum of the parts. We human beings, for example; you can't know who we are, what we are like, by simply describing our organs, bones, facial expressions, or even our personalities. You can't present a spreadsheet with data about yourself and transmit anything important at all about who you are as a person. It wasn't yet clear to me that it was my propensity to use deductive reasoning to pull apart who I was that was actually limiting a deep understanding of myself. Either I was a label—*adventure writer*—and an adjective—*successful*—or I was my diagnosis, *a sick person*, a *failure*. I deconstructed myself, diminished myself, abused myself, limited myself, and allowed others to do it to me, and I was tired. If I could have told myself that one day, decades later, I'd find myself standing at the foot of Shiva Mountain renouncing it all, promising not to deconstruct myself any longer, and finally love *me*. . . . I couldn't see it yet. A road may go somewhere, but where was mine headed?

It would be many years before I got there. The jungle was still so thick around me, so loud, dense, and frightening. Had I even found the first stone on the road out? At this point in my life, I was taking a lot of medications. The side effects were devastating. My hand tremors had grown worse. Most concerning was a new trend: After a reporting trip lasting a couple of weeks, I wouldn't be able to get over the jet lag, ending up in extreme day-night reversal. Then I'd end up in a depression, unable to write for weeks.

I was terrified that my editors would find out about my mental health issues and my drug use. I was terrified of messing up on assignments and then suffering the common consequence of being put out to pasture as a writer. I'd seen it happen when I was an editor. For unexplained reasons, a writer would stop producing good copy, or they'd lose their temper, or they'd disappear during a rewrite and never show up again. The editors would shrug, shake their heads, and stop sending them work. I was driven by fear that I would become one of them: I'd be blackballed or I'd disappear. If I wasn't a writer, if that wasn't my status, what was I?

So now, thank God, *Wired* had called and India was calling—there was still work for me. I flew there via LA and Singapore in late July and I spent my first two weeks inside the corporate headquarters of major Indian tech companies—Wipro, Tata, and Infosys. I spent evenings interviewing engineers, project managers, investors, and executives in swanky restaurants and bars, where women in short shorts and crop tops served drinks and lit the male clientele's cigars. Maybe success was still in my cards.

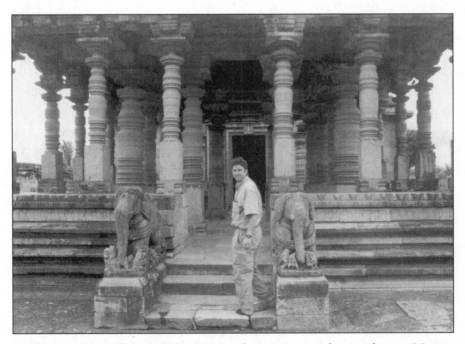

My friend Craig Collins took this picture of me as I entered a temple near Mysore, India, in 1999. The image still makes me cry.

After my last interview, I taxied back to my hotel, threw my things into my backpack, and hired a car for a few days of sightseeing. Outside Mysore, I visited an ancient temple complex devoted to Vishnu, the sustainer of the universe. I was mesmerized by the ornate carvings of elephants, goddesses, and even humans having sex in various positions. I was thrilled by the way India seemed to exist simultaneously in modern and medieval times. Cars, trucks, and ox carts shared the roads. Men and women worked in fields next to factories. I felt a holiness stirring inside me in India, which I hesitate to say because I'm aware of the fetishizing of ancient Asian and Indigenous cultures. I'm aware of the colonial trappings of spiritual seeking and travel writing. *Western bro has spiritual experience while traveling in impoverished countries.* And yet, it is my experience that India does have special qualities that can be felt, if you choose to pay attention. As one Indian yoga teacher I later met with explained: matter and spirit are more combined in India. Swamis and yogis I've met there have suggested to me that the subcontinent's people have been working with spiritual technologies for thousands of years. Maybe it's in the soil itself.

After Mysore, I flew to Varanasi, formerly Banaras. Located on the Ganges, Varanasi is one of the world's most ancient cities and is regarded as one of its holiest. Indians travel to Varanasi at the end of life, believing that if one dies there, one stands a better chance of leaving karma and samsara—the cycle of suffering, death, and rebirth—behind. The hope is to avoid being reincarnated again, instead achieving *moksha*, liberation, and becoming one with the spiritual realm.

By the time I arrived in Varanasi, I was feeling a hunger for more spiritual and less journalistic tourism. In the temples near Mysore, I felt a holiness that I never felt at home. I wanted more of it, and I thought, perhaps understandably, that it must come from these places—that it was external, entering from the outside, a filling up rather than a filling in. I'd later come to understand that feelings of connection, even holiness, originate inside us. It is, as the saying goes, an inside job. But at the time,

I assumed that this feeling came from the walls of the temples, from the holy sites themselves, from the air and the soil of these transporting places. And I wanted more.

I traveled to the Deer Park in Sarnath, where the Buddha delivered his first sermon to his followers. The grove reminded me of the scene in *Siddhartha*, my favorite book, in which Siddhartha, a spiritual seeker suffering from the confusion of his childhood, meets the Buddha in a grove in the village of Savathi. Siddhartha had traveled for years, seeking wisdom from gurus, when he and his friend Govind realize that, in the Buddha, they've met a truly realized being. The Buddha had awakened to the truth and was enlightened. So, Govind chooses to become a disciple. But Siddhartha asks for a meeting with the Buddha. He confronts him on the flaws of his method. He gets right up in the Buddha's face—politely, but still in his face. Then he says farewell to Govind and the Buddha. He realizes that he cannot submit to another man's system of thought, even if it's a perfect system. He must find his way to the truth on his own, or he must die trying.

Somehow, this passage, as well as a passage from *The Razor's Edge*, when Larry meets with Sri Ganesh and experiences the presence of an enlightened being, became inextricably linked to my story. To my romantic way of thinking, India and I seemed karmically entangled. I'd read the books in high school, but suddenly these quotes were alive inside me. This passage shakes me up every time I read it: the image of Siddhartha walking away from the Buddha. The image, in *The Razor's Edge*, of Larry walking away from his Western life and everybody's expectations of him and living as a seeker in India, seemed to grip my very soul.

I took a taxi into Varanasi. I walked past men without legs, blind beggars, people who appeared to have leprosy or something like it. I walked down the steps, called *ghats*, to the Ganges, and I soaked my feet in it. I remembered something a cabdriver in Bangalore had said to me: "If you want to feel alive, you've got to see the bodies burn." So, I hired a boat to take me a few miles upriver to the Manikarnika—the burning ghat.

When we arrived, the young Indian boatman, chatty, wiry, and strong, maneuvered our skiff against the pier. I stepped out onto the powdery riverbank and into a totally different world, part daydream, part nightmare.

I climbed the stairs into a cloud of acrid smoke that covered the sun and clogged my lungs. I found my footing a few feet away from a hot pyre. It took a minute for my eyes to work out exactly what I was looking at: a corpse in the final stages of cremation. Well, not the entire corpse—only a pelvis, two partial femurs, the backbone, and a blackened bulb in a state of half-collapse remained. But it was the skull with fire shooting from the eye sockets and mouth that stole my attention. *Whose skull was this? Where had they lived? How long did they live? How did they die? What did their life amount to?* My internal questions came quick as my journalist self tried to process what I was seeing.

I felt a lump in my throat. My chest ached at the finality. This human being's time was up. This incarnation played out. The bag of bones and skin going up in flames. What I was seeing was holy, both beautiful because it was so true, and also terrifying for that same reason. And then I wanted different answers: *Who had they loved? Where were they now? How were they grieving? How were they dealing with the human-sized hole in their lives?*

Then anxious thoughts shifted me out of my reverie. *This is too intimate. I shouldn't be here.* I glanced at the firekeeper and gestured my doubts. He saw me, and then kept working. He added more wood and stoked the fire with a long, metal pole. I concluded that I was there as a witness—to the mystery and to his part in it.

Eventually, the body disappeared, transformed by heat and time into ash, smoke, and nothingness. But the firekeeper knew that more needed to be done. He stirred the ashes with the long rod until he found something solid. I couldn't see what it was. He paraded it down the stairs and set it on a small boat decorated with flowers and a lit candle. Then he picked up the boat and, setting it on the water, pushed it into the river.

Silently, I watched this blackened vertebra take its final journey onto the Ganges, where it joined other floating offerings on their final journeys. At first, I gazed only at my offering, but soon I became aware of the hundreds of candlelit offerings on the river. Together, they formed a loose-knit fleet. The many became one. And the lit candles merged with the flickering lights emanating from the city on the riverbank. The light of living and the dead. One.

I said a silent prayer for all, and then I climbed back into the boat and sat quietly as my chatty boat driver delivered me back to Varanasi's city center. There, I picked up where I'd left off: gawking at religious temples, eating chicken tikka masala, and talking to strangers. I felt both sleepy and anxious at the same time, so I popped a Dexedrine and a lorazepam. I walked until I came to a dilapidated building of gray and black stone. *Sadhus* gathered out front and entered and exited. I asked a stranger what temple it was. "Shiva."

I didn't know much about Shiva then, the god of destruction and rebirth, but I knew I had to go inside. I was utterly compelled. I stepped from the chaos of the street into the temple. It was dark and smoky, too dark to see much more than the shapes of *sadhus* crouching, bowing, lying down on the filthy floor. *Sadhus* are wandering holy men devoted to Shiva. They wear their beards long and decorate them with orange-red power. The temple reverberated with their susurration to Shiva, who is seen as being pure consciousness. A wildly unpredictable god. Were these men in the temple holy or insane? They seemed to be both.

In the front of the chamber was a phallic stone, coated in an oily mess that I later learned was ghee, which has the same consistency as butter. I spent a good thirty minutes in the temple, trying to absorb the energy of the place and the men in it. I wanted what they had. No, not the insanity. I sort of had that already. I wanted the devotion. I wanted to believe in something greater than me. I was hungry to live a different life. Could I be a *sadhu*? No. But maybe I could be a spiritual person again?

As I sat in the corner of the Shiva temple, taking in the sights, sounds, smells, and the powerful energy, I thought about my love of and devotion to Jesus as a kid. I read the Bible and prayed daily. I meditated on Jesus. I was a total Jesus freak. I considered myself a little mystic. Remember the mystical merging experiences that I told Dr. Jerry about? I wanted more of those. And now, in that temple, I wanted *out*. I wanted out of the straitjacket of a success-seeking writer fueled by external affirmations that would never be enough. I wanted out of pretense and into depth and authenticity. I was another greedy American chasing fame and fortune, destined to have a midlife crisis. Thank God I didn't have kids, or I'd be messing them up something fierce. Thank God Di hadn't left me yet, because I deserved that, too.

After half an hour in the temple, I walked out and hailed a cab. Back in my hotel room, I ordered room service but didn't eat. I fell asleep with chicken tikka masala and a mango lassi, still my favorite meal, on the table, which wasn't like me. I slept through the night and through the next day. I woke up at dusk, confused as to where I was. I scrambled to the bathroom to find my satchel of pills and took two of each. I feared that the intensity and fatigue would lead me into another depression. I fell asleep again.

The next morning, I tried unsuccessfully to shit for the third straight day and couldn't. Damn, the Dexedrine has stopped up my gut again. I checked out of the hotel, caught a cab to the airport, flew to Delhi, switched planes, and flew back to the States. When I got back to my house, I held Di. I told her all about my experience, but I could tell she didn't understand. I began writing the piece the next day but found I didn't care about the subject—the tech industry—anymore. When I got to the ending, I had nothing to say. I called my friend Andrew and asked him to help me write the ending. He took a stab at it. I pasted in what he'd written and sent the article off to Alex. It wasn't my best work, but it didn't stink up the joint, either.

Then I received a letter from *George*. They were terminating my contract. I had bonked an article, and they asked me to send them my notes, which were so disorganized that even I couldn't read them. They were done with me. I was done with me. I pulled the shades down and fell into a depression unlike any I'd had before. For three months, I barely left the house.

What had started it? The jet lag, the ceaseless medication, getting the boot from *George*, a spiritual crisis. The reasons didn't matter because I believed I couldn't fix them. Everything in the living world paled next to the burning ghat. I wanted to go back. I wanted to watch more bodies burn. I never recovered from that India trip. Not just physically but emotionally. I didn't want to be an adventure writer anymore. I didn't want to please editors. I wanted to write about what I felt and saw and experienced. The burning was all that mattered. The burning made me feel alive. I would burn all of it—everything—down.

I CAN'T EVEN arrange these years in a way that makes narrative sense. I have little memory of what I did. My altar now is covered with tchotchkes from thirty countries that stir memories from distant places, but they don't form a coherent story. I was too foggy at the time to store the memories in a clear way.

Except for the burning ghat. For the longest time, my memories of that place served as a spiritual anchor. I sought experiences like it. I thought going places and experiencing things would show me a way to live more spiritually. I wanted to learn about myself, but I believed that the wisdom was out there, in the world, in a temple, in a guru, in an intense experience. If only I could go to enough places. See enough of it. Someday, it would resonate, it would all make sense. And my loneliness would disappear.

Eventually the depression lifted a bit, and I picked up some assignments again. In Manaus, Brazil, a jungle city along the Amazon River about nine hundred miles inland from the Atlantic, I went to a witch doctor to diagnose my marriage. He sold me a black, phallic-shaped candle and told me to light it when my wife and I had sex. In Bali, I went to a holy woman. She told me to pray to Kali Ma, the Mother of All. Everywhere, I looked for examples, to turn them into lessons. Where was the next Gene Savoy to show me how to find a road?

And this was maddening, not only to me but to the people in my life. "Why are you doing this, Brad? What are you searching for?"

Chasing. I was chasing messiahs.

I was chasing my father, desperate for him to reach out to me as I was drowning in the river in Arkansas. Instead, he was motionless and did nothing but stare down at me.

In the summer of 2001, feeling another depression coming on, I begged Dr. Winston, a handsome youthful psychiatrist I'd begun seeing shortly after I moved to Santa Fe, to do something more radical. He had two suggestions. The first: electro-convulsant therapy, shock therapy. The second: add an antipsychotic medication, Zyprexa, to my already sizable cocktail of meds. I chose the latter. Within two months, I gained thirty-five pounds, and, worse, I felt like a zombie, one who lives on ten bowls of cereal a day. The meds caused me to make mistakes that were getting noticed. I would leave my day pack at a security checkpoint or a notebook in a restaurant. In addition to the prescription drugs, I was self-medicating with alcohol and caffeine. I drank coffee when I felt low and beer when I felt too jagged from the Dexedrine. I had become an addict, and more than that, as my nervous system frayed under the drugs, it became more important than ever that I save my career. I couldn't imagine a life in which I wasn't a successful magazine writer. I couldn't imagine what I'd do. I'd be a nobody. I'd be useless. This was my greatest fear.

The antipsychotic succeeded in smoothing out the jagged nervousness that was making me feel so ungrounded and angry. Now I was chill, but the problem was I couldn't feel anything. Everything about my body felt numb, including my brain. No longer did words playfully ricochet around in my head, an experience I had identified as the source of my creativity. It's what fueled my writing and made it a little different. And now, I couldn't feel it.

I began the twenty-first century descending further and further into hell. But I took another trip, this one to the Czech Republic to write for *Outside* about dilettante tramps, everyday men and women with decent jobs who spent their leisure time dressing up like Depression-era hobos or American cowboys and Indians.

On the flight over I had a flashback and a panic attack. I was at the dinner table, calling out my drunk father and looking over to my mom and siblings for support. Nothing but angry stares. I was sitting next to my father's drunk body, hating myself, terrified that he was going to die. All I could think about was grabbing the handle of the plane's cabin door, pulling it, and jumping out the window. I tugged on the arm of a flight attendant and told her. She simply said, "That would kill all of us." I sank back into my seat and gripped the chair.

When I arrived in the Prague airport, I immediately bought a ticket on the next flight to the States. At home, I called my editor, who talked me into trying again. I restocked on lorazepam, flew back to Europe, spent three weeks with the "hobos," and somehow completed the story. Somehow, I took another trip, this time to Italy, to write about mountaineer Reinhold Messner. Somehow, I wrote those stories while hopped up on Dexedrine, lorazepam, and antipsychotics. And the next year, travel writer Paul Theroux chose my hobo story for the *Best American Travel Writing* anthology. *Outside* chose my Czech Republic tramping story for its *Outside 25: Classic Tales and New Voices from the Frontiers of Adventure* collection. That should have made me happy, made me proud, but I knew that my career was over. Not only couldn't I do the work anymore, but I also didn't really want to. Was it the antipsychotics that stole my joy, or was my lack of joy the reason I needed the antipsychotics? I don't know. When yet another depression arrived, and they always arrived, I switched to another antipsychotic, Risperdal. I stood in front of the mirror and watched myself take this new drug.

That night, I drove an hour to see the spiritual teacher Ram Dass give a talk, and when I got home, I felt the drug taking hold. I took a lorazepam, a sleeping pill, and another Risperdal. The next thing I knew, it was 3 p.m. the following day. A friend was sitting in the kitchen.

"Why are you here?"

"Di asked me to watch over you. She was concerned. She had to go to work. But she wants you to call her."

When the Twin Towers fell a few weeks later, I slept through it. Di tried calling five or six times before I finally answered.

"Did you see what happened in New York?"

"No, what?"

Eventually, I completely lost my ability to keep up with my work. I took on a natural history column in *Outside*, which I wrote poorly. I did a few stories during the next four or five years, but not very many. And they didn't go smoothly. I didn't tell any of my friends or colleagues that I was barely leaving my house. The calls were getting fewer and further between. Or maybe I wasn't even talking to editors anymore. Di and I kept my state a secret. When I look back at pictures from that time, you might not see it, but I see it. I'm puffy. My eyes are vacant. I kept a shotgun in the closet of my home office.

In 2005, *Outside* called and asked if I'd spend two weeks driving a car around Nevada and then write a road trip story about it. I consented. I fought the fog and managed to hike, kayak, rock climb, and more. But, admittedly, I spent far more time sleeping in my hotel rooms.

In 2006, GQ called and asked whether I had any story ideas. I didn't, but after a quick Google search, I pitched a story about fundamentalist missionary surfers from Hawaii who traveled to Indonesia to try to convert Muslims from what they considered a counterfeit religion.

A week later, I was on a plane to Indonesia. I still took the same massive cocktail of antipsychotics, mood stabilizers, antidepressants, sedatives, amphetamines, sleeping pills, and more. On a hike with the surfers, I collapsed in the jungle in Lombok. I spent forty-eight hours in bed, getting up to pee every fifteen or twenty minutes. I downplayed that something was wrong. "I just need to rest," I told the surfers. Something was clearly very wrong, but I was too exhausted to care.

I eventually pulled myself out of bed to join them for a boat ride to Bali for a dinner outing. I put on a shirt and shorts and sandals. When it was my turn to step from the boat to a dinghy to take us to shore, I missed the dinghy and stepped right into the clear, cold ocean. As I descended, I waited for the familiar feeling of the water catching me like it does when you jump into a swimming pool's deep end. I waited for that feeling when your momentum slows and then stops and then you feel the water lifting you up, supporting you, assuring you that it wants to carry you back to the surface where you can breathe. But I felt none of this. Even physics and Mother Earth seemed to be done with me. I'm sure I was imagining this, but I swear my downward momentum increased, as if the center of the earth was pulling me farther down . . . down, down, down. And, you know what? I didn't care.

As I sunk down into the water, I felt a deep sense of relief. Why relief? Why not embarrassment that I had just walked into the ocean and would need to be pulled out by the surfers? As I felt myself falling toward the ocean floor, I knew I had reached the nadir. For a few seconds, I let my body relax, sink into the water. I could feel the gasp of air I'd taken when I fell draining from my lungs. My dream to be a successful writer was over. It had been over for a while. My drug-fueled groping for fame was over, and it was time to let go. I opened my eyes under the water, but all I saw was the gun in my closet. It was underneath the wool blanket. It was not any gun; it was a sawed-off shotgun I'd purchased at a garage sale in Santa Fe.

Perhaps it was time to put it to its intended purpose.

The surfers fished me out of the ocean. Heavy. Wet. I was alive, I guess.

eleven

THE END OF THE DREAM

W HEN I RETURNED TO SANTA FE, I HAD A TERRIBLE UPPER-respiratory infection in addition to my peeing problem, which had eased to once every hour. I showed up at my local urgent care and a doctor ordered blood work. The results showed very high protein levels in my blood. My kidneys were shutting down. I made an appointment with my internist, who referred me immediately to a nephrologist. He ordered more tests and shared his theory.

"Your decade and a half on lithium, combined with your dehydration in the jungle of Lombok, has poisoned your kidneys."

He wasn't sure how bad the damage was, but he had sobering news about kidney damage from lithium toxicity—it typically doesn't bounce back. Sometimes long-term dialysis is necessary. Di slumped in her chair and cried. He ordered more tests and said one of the worst things a doctor can say: "We will have to wait to see."

I didn't rest. I couldn't rest. An editor at GQ, with whom I'd shared nothing about my travails in Indonesia, was waiting for my story. I spent the next week writing the surfing article, while filling plastic jugs with pee and writing down the exact times of each evacuation. This was not the sexy writer's life I had planned for myself. And my editor didn't like my first draft.

Every few weeks, I returned to the nephrologist to receive updates, hoping and praying that my blood-protein scores would return to levels close to normal and that I would begin to pee less frequently.

I wrote a second draft, and my editor still wasn't happy. I wrote third, fourth, fifth, sixth, and seventh drafts. In the end, he accepted the piece and paid me, but I clearly wasn't writing with my same verve and lucidity.

Once the story had gone to bed, I did too. I shuffled between my bed and the couch, watching CNN by day and baseball by night. I didn't bother pitching story ideas. I felt embarrassed that I wasn't writing. I told my friends I was "working on a book proposal." Di and I spent evenings on opposite sides of our house. The emotional distance between us was growing. We barely touched each other. There was no animosity, just a drifting apart. We didn't discuss our relationship much. When my psychiatrist suggested that I apply for government disability, Di and I worked on the application together. A few months later, I received news that I qualified due to my severe depression and the deeply debilitating effects of the medications I needed to take to control it.

I would wake at noon, walk to the nearest cafe, and try to make sense of the *New York Times*. I carried a stack of magazines with me, but I rarely made it through an entire feature in the same magazines that, a few years ago, I had cover stories in. When GQ ran my surfer story, I didn't even read it.

In fact, I rarely read my articles once they appeared in print. I feared seeing typos or bigger mistakes, or writing that seemed less skillful than I believed I was capable of. In other words: I didn't read my articles because I feared I wasn't perfect. Moreover, I feared that I would see how vapid or meaningless travel stories were in the end. My articles were entertainment, and while we editors and writers viewed *Outside* as somehow culturally significant, it was just a self-righteous permutation of *Entertainment* or *People*. It was a magazine about hiking and mountain biking, hobbies popular with rich people. My articles were little more than content, a necessary thing so that the ad department could sell full-page display advertisements to car manufacturers and high-end sportswear companies. To what end? *Outside*'s owner, Larry Burke, was a volatile CEO whose shouting echoed down the hallways. Writers complained to me that it often took months, sometimes a year, for Burke's accountants to pay them. After we published "Into Thin Air," Larry came into my office with a look betraying anger and worry.

"The article ran at seventeen thousand words," Larry complained. "Do we have to pay him for it all?"

Really? I thought. Our writer had almost died getting that story, was now dealing with the death of his compatriots, and Larry's concern was the money. Given my upbringing around aggressive men who gaslit, Larry elicited a dark, soulless feeling in my body. I looked up from the papers I was reading and stared at him. "Yes," was all I said, and I returned to my reading.

And now, lying on my couch with the curtains drawn against the sun, as heavily medicated as I could manage and still breathe, my thoughts circled obsessively around my ten-year run as a freelance adventure writer. In my twenties and thirties, it seemed so elemental to who I was. First, it was the only thing I knew how to do. I traveled. I told stories. And through that process, I filtered reality and made sense of my life. Second, I loved it and couldn't imagine any other career. But now? My entire journey as a writer, and the ambition that fueled it, seemed laughable. Misguided. Cruel to Di. Maybe even cruel to myself.

I had pushed myself so hard—and for what? I'd carried backpacks full of pills all over the world. It hadn't occurred to me that my tendency to forget or misplace important items was a sign that this way of life wasn't working, or that I should find a new calling. It only made me work harder. I would castigate myself for being so mindless and create obsessive routines and checklists. But even with these supposed failsafe routines in place, I remained a walking shit show, leaving day packs, notebooks, jackets, phones all over the countries I moved through, hoping I wouldn't yet again hear my name over the airport PA system: "Paging Mr. Brad Wetzler, paging Mr. Wetzler. Please return to the security desk to retrieve your backpack full of medications."

Looking back, I was a man without a coherent story about himself, about his childhood, about his father—and so I wrote about others' successes and triumphs in an attempt to create my own. The Dalai Lama reportedly once said, "The reason romantic relationships are so difficult is because they are an attempt to join reality with fantasy." I loved Di. But travel writing had grown into a romantic partner, too. And I was struggling to marry the reality of my life with the fantasy of my dream job.

I didn't understand this then, but so much of my drive was a misguided attempt to please an impossible father. It was an unconscious strategy to say, *Hey, Dad. Look at me. See how smart and successful I am? See how I'm even getting close to semi-famous? Will you love me now? Please?*

Not only was I trying to play the game of pleasing my own patriarch; I worked to fit into our cultural patriarchal paradigm too—to become successful by cultural standards where money and status are expected. A world where a man who makes a decent living working as a schoolteacher or a tradesman has less status than a stockbroker making big bucks.

In my early fifties, while submitting to twice-weekly therapy sessions, my therapist suggested I had an *internal father complex*, an inner split. Instead of having a single internal father figure, I had two. One was an idealized version of my father as the charismatic, highly intelligent lawyer I would stop at virtually nothing trying to please.

The other was a more honest version of the father I'd grown up with. This father had abandoned me for alcohol, verbally demeaned me, lied to me, gaslit me, and betrayed me. This version was the father who came to dinner drunk, whom I walked to bed afterward, who hurt my mother with his ongoing affair, who forced me into impossible situations in which I had to comfort her. This father damaged our family, causing me decades of suffering and depression. This internal version of my father had caused me to take prescription drugs until my kidneys failed. How did I feel about him? I hated him with a passion. In twenty-five years of traveling, in twenty-five years of seeking, taking drugs, going to therapy, chasing sex and love and messiahs of all shapes and forms, I failed to heal this split.

IN 2008, DR. WINSTON TOLD ME ABOUT A NEW ANTIPSYCHOTIC THAT supposedly had fewer debilitating side effects than Risperdal, Zyprexa, or Seroquel, all of which I'd taken: Abilify. I told him I wanted to try it. Within three months, my mind became less foggy. I felt more emotions. Parts of me that had been too numb to participate in my life came back online. I no longer felt like I had cotton stuffed into my brain and nervous system. Instead of sleeping till noon, I began to wake before dawn. I read. I wrote. Most striking, I had a libido for the first time in almost seven years. I longed for touch. I craved sex.

But Di and I had forgotten how to even hold each other. Had I been so self-centered, so singularly driven to become successful, that I'd turned my marriage into little more than a support system for my ambition? We started seeing a couple's therapist, though it was increasingly clear that we were headed for divorce.

Meanwhile, I began flirting with women in an online chatroom. Eventually, I began an affair. I returned home after, too ashamed to continue to be married. As soon as I walked in the door, I confessed. I told Di I thought I should move out. The next day, I rented an apartment. I couldn't live with myself as a cheater. Staying with Di would have made me too much like my father. Just like that, I abandoned my wife and best friend of fifteen years to avoid becoming my dad. Today, Di and I are friends, but I am still deeply ashamed of my impulsive, awful behavior.

And yet—as much as it may sound like a rationalization—I knew. I knew that I was facing a long journey of healing and that I had to face it alone. I was still a teenager who needed to grow up, but I also felt like an old sage who had already learned a great deal about suffering and the deeper meaning of life. I craved disappearing to a cave in the Himalayas.

So, much lay ahead of me. And it couldn't happen in our marriage.

The first months of my new life as a single man were rough. After a few months, I ended the affair. I dated and slept with many women — one-night stands, weeklong and monthlong mini-relationships that were lit, flared, and then fizzled in rapid succession. And then a friend introduced me to Andrea, a smart, sexy sculptor who'd grown up in Santa Fe. She claimed to be descended from Russian royalty; created beautiful, brooding assemblage sculptures; and collected antiques. I was instantly in love. Of course. We became inseparable. I was kidding myself that I was ready for a relationship. After only four months of dating, I moved into her antique-stuffed, Alice in Wonderland–like home. We barely left the house. It felt like refuge from the storm.

I was no longer a working journalist. I felt too numbed out, too foggy, and when I tried to write, I couldn't get past the first paragraph. I obsessively wrote and rewrote it. Besides, the internet had destroyed the pay model. I was living on government disability checks. Andrea taught me how to pick out valuable objects at garage sales. We opened a booth at the flea market. I had gone from world-traveling writer to overmedicated shut-in to junk dealer. I'd buy a wooden coatrack for twenty dollars and sell it as an antique at the flea market for thirty. It didn't occur to me that this wasn't going to work out, financially or romantically. I felt more alive than I had in years. And I was going with the feelings. I loved Andrea, the sex was good, and I had hope that things would get better.

A few months after I moved in, I learned that the melanoma that had first appeared in my mother's left eye five years earlier was spreading rapidly throughout her body. I soon became close friends with Paul, Andrea's thirty-year-old nephew. He was smart, intelligent, and, like me, taking massive quantities of medications for depression or bipolar disorder. Paul lived with his mother, Andrea's sister, Sylvie. We met weekly at her kitchen table and discussed the writings of C. G. Jung, especially the *Red Book*, his weird, mystical notebook in which he explored his unconscious and tried to make sense of his own mental struggles through drawing and writing.

One day, Paul looked up from his coffee and told me he was going to attempt to make sense of his life in a notebook like the *Red Book*. He would write, doodle, and think his way out of his predicament.

"Brad, these drugs have killed my spirit. If I fail in my *Black Book*, I plan to kill my body, too."

Years later, I am filled with sorrow and shame about my weak reaction to his statement: "I hear you, Paul. I don't blame you. I hope you figure it out, and, if not, I understand."

Two months later, I was in bed with Andrea at 5 a.m. when the phone rang. Andrea answered. I knew what had happened by the tone of her voice. "We will be right there."

I followed Andrea into the house, hugged Sylvie, and made my way over to Paul's still, blue body stretched out on the hallway floor. The police detectives and the coroner were busying themselves with the chores of working a suicide.

I sat down next to Paul, who was naked except for white briefs. I set my hand over his heart. I said a silent prayer. I cried, tears that had seemingly formed in the pit of my stomach. Then I sat at the kitchen table, where we'd met so often, and joined family and friends in talking about what a kind, confused soul Paul had been. We talked about the abuse he suffered as a child at the hands of a pedophile. We talked about the failures of the psychiatric industry and its ironic addiction to believing that drugs are the only answer to mental health problems.

The coroner asked me to help put Paul's body into the body bag. We spread the orange, nylon bag on the carpet next to him. I grabbed Paul's feet while the coroner grabbed his arms. We lifted him up and set him inside the bag. I zipped it up to his chest, and the coroner pulled the zipper over his face. As Paul disappeared into the orange cocoon, I felt sorrow and relief for him. Sorrow at his short, tragic life; relief that his suffering was over.

I helped lift Paul onto the gurney, and the coroner and I wheeled him to the hearse waiting in the driveway. As I watched them pull away, I felt a stirring in my gut that I hadn't felt in years. It had been so long it almost felt new. I don't know how to describe it except to say that it felt like a part of me that had my own best interest at heart blinked open its eyes after a long, long sleep. And for the first time I sensed a primal urge to save myself, to protect myself, to do what was necessary to move forward in my life. And just maybe, to heal.

I told Andrea and Sylvie that I needed to go home to nap, but that I'd be back in a while. Back at Andrea's house, I lay down and wept at my inner emptiness and the mess of my life. I felt lost at sea. That deep urge for self-preservation, to value my own life, didn't go away. But I doubted whether, at age forty-seven, I had the guts, stamina, and time left to pull off a self-reclamation attempt. I was not arrogant enough to think that saving myself would be quick or easy.

The next months passed by slowly. There was no reason for joy in Andrea's and my life. We seemed powerless, as if we were both drowning in deep, black water. We were both thrashing about for a life preserver, but all we had to hold onto was each other.

And then, one day, while writing in my journal about my childhood obsession with Jesus, I had an idea. The previous night I'd read an article about a newly minted walking trail in northern Israel that followed the path that Jesus may have followed when he left his home of Nazareth and went to the Sea of Galilee to begin his three-year ministry. Those three years altered the spiritual and political history of Western civilization. The path was called the Jesus Trail.

I closed my journal, went to my computer, and dashed out a story pitch to an editor at the *New York Times* I'd written travel articles for—many years ago. I proposed to walk the Jesus Trail and write a personal narrative for the Travel page. She wrote back a few hours later: "Go."

This felt different and new. Yes, I was deciding to write another story, but this time, it was for me, and it mattered. My article wasn't going to sell magazine ads; it was going to move people. This time it was for spirit and inspiration and a step toward that holiness I'd felt in India and maybe hadn't felt since.

I logged onto a travel booking website and bought a plane ticket to Tel Aviv, leaving in forty-eight hours. I skulked downstairs where Andrea was resting to tell her my plans.

"I'm going to Israel on Sunday to write a travel story. I will be gone a while."

"How long?"

"I'm not sure, sweetie. I doubt I'll be back for a month."

On Sunday morning, a taxi picked me up at 5 a.m., and I rode in silence to the Albuquerque airport. I boarded a plane and popped a sleeping pill and a lorazepam. Twenty-four hours later, I woke up in the Holy Land. I deplaned, traded dollars for shekels, and rented a car. I had $3,000 dollars to my name and no return ticket. *I can't get into* that *much trouble with such a small amount of money,* I thought, as I drove across Israel's green coastal plain toward Galilee.

I parked my car behind a gas station in the dark in downtown Nazareth. I spotted a sign for the Old City. I hauled my backpack onto my shoulders, shrugged to adjust the weight, and strolled through dark, narrow, stone streets past houses built more than a thousand years ago. Fifteen minutes later, I arrived at the gate of a hostel where I'd booked a room.

"Hi, I'm Brad, the travel writer for the *New York Times.*"

The clerk smiled and welcomed me. He showed me my room. I tossed my backpack in the corner and collapsed on the bed. I don't remember what I was thinking that night. I was too tired. But I suspect I felt something like, *What a long, strange trip this has been.* I quickly fell asleep.

I woke the next morning, threw on the same shorts and shirt that had served me well on assignments all over the world, and ate breakfast in the hostel's small cafe.

I headed out the door, map in hand, to find the spot where the trail's founder had agreed to meet me a few days before. He graciously introduced me to a couple of twentysomething guides he had hired to lead me on the four-day hike, during which we planned to cover the forty miles of the Jesus Trail.

We stepped out of the courtyard, and that's when I noticed the trailhead—just two words painted in orange on the wall of the building: Jesus Trail. An arrow pointed to the right. I gazed in the direction of the arrow. All I saw were steps leading uphill. Hundreds, thousands, of vertical steps. The path out of Nazareth and into the next chapter of my life. There was little doubt about the first steps of my quest to reclaim my body, my mind, my life. This journey, this work to excavate my soul would be an uphill, sacred battle.

I nodded to the guides, tightened the straps on my pack, and took the first step.

twelve

RUNNING TOWARD, RUNNING AWAY

WAS CLIMBING THE STEEP STEPS THROUGH NAZARETH'S OLD
City, along streets so narrow I couldn't see the sky. The steps were un-
evenly spaced. One long stride reached some, while others required two
or three mini-steps and a skip. I struggled to find a groove. And there
were so many pleasant distractions: sights, smells, and sounds. I passed
dim cafes buzzing with the chatter of old, bearded men sipping strong,
Arab-style coffee and spice shops so completely full of colorful powders—
bright yellows, reds, burnt umbers, even blacks—that a person couldn't
even enter to shop. I kept walking, climbing, sweating, breathing. The
crisp, 50-degree air cooled my lungs, but I couldn't get enough of it,
and so I paused to desperately reach for my breath—head down, hands
on hips, inhaling as deeply as I could. But, step by step, I made slow
progress.

I would need a steady pace to complete the forty-mile Jesus Trail
over the next four days. I knew at my deepest level that I wasn't just
hiking a trail; I was stepping into the rest of my life. I was aware that I
needed to write a new and very different next chapter for myself. I was
also acutely aware that I didn't know how, and I was afraid. How could I
possibly transform into someone who could live and thrive without being

numbed out? Being present felt terrifying, but I knew there was no other option if I wanted to live at all. I might have to find a new way to make a living. I'd have to finally learn how to be in close, intimate relationship with friends and, I hoped, a partner. I would need to be more discerning about who I allowed into my life and heart. I wasn't sure if Andrea and I would make it. It was overwhelming and made my heart pick up its pounding in my chest.

But if my heart rate was increasing, time itself felt like it was slowing down. I felt more present with the world and myself, like I was dropping in. Into what? Into the life I was supposed to live. Or maybe I was falling out of the life I wasn't supposed to be living. Maybe I wasn't meant to be a travel writer. Maybe I was meant to simply heal. Eventually, I settled down. My breathing evened out. I put my hand on my heart and felt. Just felt. And when I did, the chaos within and without slowed down. I actually noticed things. Real things. Wholesome things, like humans connecting with each other with kindness. I noticed the gentle smile of an elderly shopkeeper. Was she really smiling at me? I heard children laughing. I saw a couple holding each other in a warm, loving embrace. This was a world I hadn't paid much attention to lately. Was I seeing goodness? What about inside me? Did I contain goodness? Maybe I wasn't half bad. I encouraged myself to pay more attention to the ways the world is NOT broken.

And, man, it felt great to be traveling again after years of living in-doors, hyper-medicated, practically homebound. And while I was there to write a story for the *New York Times*, I wasn't there to please them, and that was a new, unfamiliar feeling. I didn't need the clip. I'd written so many articles in my fifteen years as a travel editor and writer that one more story on my resume wasn't going to do anything big for me or my ego. I was here now for me. I was here because I loved the subject and wanted to learn about where Jesus lived and walked, and what he might have been doing. In learning more about Jesus, I also wanted to learn more about myself and why my childhood interest in this prophet was so intense and ardent. Jesus was a bright, sacred spot that glowed through the murky mess of my childhood memories. And, most importantly, I was here because I wanted to live.

I was in the Holy Land for many reasons that felt authentic and right. The way my body was responding was confirming this. With each step, I noticed an invitation to be present to my surroundings. I was aware of my feet and felt the earth underneath my shoes. It felt firm, supportive, grounding. The Mediterranean air in my lungs felt fresh and crisp. I was ready to stop betraying myself—with drugs, with people pleasing, with chasing success.

I knew that I had far to go and that walking in Jesus's footsteps for a few days, however challenging and fascinating, would not fix me or make me feel whole. I would not go from selling junk at the flea market to being successful in some new career, and I couldn't magically walk away from my depression and loneliness.

After an hour of slogging up the steps, absorbing the electric aliveness of this small, busy city, I reached the last step and topped out on a busy throughway. The sky opened into a broad blue canvas dotted with puffy cumulus clouds. Cars, taxis, and small trucks zoomed by. At a crosswalk, I pressed the Walk button on a light pole and waited for the signal to change. My legs ached from the climbing, but I could honestly say the ache felt good. Sort of. I looked out across the green cow pastures and spotted the tan line of the trail—that's where I was headed. As an excuse to catch my breath, I pulled my Jesus Trail map out of my pack and looked it over.

The trail crossed the region known as Galilee, by turns green and rolling and mountainous and rocky, traditionally believed to be the birthplace of Jesus of Nazareth. The trail headed north to Zippori National Park and then through the Arab village of Mash'had and east toward Cana, where Jesus turned water into wine at a wedding, one of his most-cited miracles. Next, it headed eastward through Beit Keshet Forest and on to an old army base. It passed within sight of Mt. Tabor, site of another miracle, the Transfiguration. As a kid, the Transfiguration confused me. Jesus climbs to the top of a mountain, and, as his disciples watch, he turns bright white. As an adult, I came to see the beautiful symbolism in the story. Jesus was showing his radiance. He was a man and godly. Was he suggesting to his disciples that they—and maybe all of us, too—are equally radiant and godly, if only we paused to notice?

From there, the trail joined up with an old Roman road to Damascus, the same road that a Jewish man named Saul was traveling along when he was struck by lightning, visited by the resurrected Jesus, and instantly transformed, changing his name to Paul and becoming one of the most important Christian evangelists. The trail passed by ancient synagogues where Jesus taught. It passed over the Horns of Hattin, a two-pronged mountain, site of a crucial battle of the Crusades. It passed through a modern-day kibbutz, one of the first group farms of the new nation of Israel, and a Holocaust memorial. After that, the trail climbed Mount Arbel and down the back side, past caves where Zealots hid from Romans. It dropped down past the Mount of Beatitudes to the Sea of Galilee, where according to the biblical story Jesus fed thousands from a single basket of fish and calmed a storm and walked on water. The trail wound finally to Capernaum, the hometown of two of the twelve apostles, Peter and Andrew, where Jesus taught in a synagogue during the first part of the three-year ministry that culminated in his crucifixion in Jerusalem, a death reserved by the Romans for criminals.

As I walked, I tried to meditate on the Jesus I remembered, the figure who had been so important to me as a kid and provided so much solace and refuge. I remembered staying up late, reading the Bible and praying. I prayed that my dad would stop drinking. I prayed that my mom might finally leave him. I prayed for sleep, an end to the insomnia that left me exhausted at school. I prayed for silly kid stuff, too. I remember praying hard that I would live long enough to have sex with a woman. I guess I was praying to feel connected, maybe even saved. I joined a Bible study group. I listened to *Jesus Christ Superstar* and fell in love with the character of Mary Magdalene. Jesus wasn't merely my savior; he was my friend. Looking back, my faith in Jesus was a reasonably healthy way to channel my depression and loneliness—and perhaps it protected that sacred spark of idealism and hope in me, a spark that was deeply threatened by the dysfunction and culture of lies in my family.

Was there a historical Jesus? Almost certainly, yes. What is not known, and probably can't be known, is whether he did anything like the things described in the Bible, or whether the text is an overlay of pagan and more ancient traditions that the redactors of the Bible attached to Jesus. In fact, there were many men who lived lives like Jesus. They emerged from Galilee and other regions to challenge the traditional Jewish teachings and the oppressive rule of Rome. Called Zealots, they traveled, taught, and even hid out in caves near the Sea of Galilee, where I was ultimately heading.

But it didn't matter to me whether Jesus was a proven historical figure. I just loved the story, the character, and I was fascinated that I'd been so enamored with him. Could digging more deeply into the Jesus story and walking in his footsteps lead me to excavate the less cynical and self-abusive parts of me I'd lost? Could I rediscover a new, healthy way to see spirituality and god, minus both the naivete and rigid, fundamentalist self-abuse? Could I be a Christian again, but one who saw Jesus more as a metaphor, a story, a myth? Could I connect with wonder and love again? Could I open my heart?

We need stories. We need to have a coherent story about our own lives. Here's the rest of Joan Didion's "we tell ourselves stories in order to live" quote: "We look for the sermon in the suicide, for the social or moral lesson in the murder of five. We interpret what we see, select the most workable of the multiple choices. We live entirely, especially if we are writers, by the imposition of a narrative line upon disparate images, by the 'ideas' with which we have learned to freeze the shifting phantasmagoria which is our actual experience."

The late nature writer Barry Lopez described the importance of stories this way: "Everything is held together with stories. That is all that is holding us together, stories and compassion."

Me? I needed both: a new story and a serious dose of compassion, especially the self-directed kind.

Clearly, I wanted to believe in something again—something outside of myself that would help me to know myself. But as I walked, I lost focus on my present experience, on how I wanted to use this time as inspiration for my future. Memories of childhood were creeping in. The constancy of the difficult relationship with my family—then and now. The lies, the shaming, the fights. At school, I got straight As; I was president of the student council and captain of the basketball team. I was voted Most Likely to Succeed and won Most Inspirational Student. Man, I was a pleaser extraordinaire, a pro. But none of that achievement translated into what felt like acceptance or love. At times, it seemed to earn me the opposite: isolation, shame. Or was it my fault? My frequent naming of my dad's blackout drinking. Or the time I blurted out at dinner that I knew the location of the secret apartment he kept for his romantic trysts with the neighbor woman. For better or worse, I could not abide by the false narrative that we were a perfect family. The wide canyon between appearances and truths stuck in my side like a lance. The little lies were nothing compared to the meta-lie that we were forced to embrace and tell and retell every day. That we were not merely a decent family but an extraordinary family. We were more successful, wealthy, and physically attractive than anybody we knew.

And with this veneer of perfection came many unspoken rules to follow: (1) Sharing feelings is not allowed. (2) The job of a kid is to fit into the family system, not to become himself or herself. (3) Asking for or stating the truth is not allowed. (4) Breaking these rules will get you ignored, ostracized, shut out.

The more I bristled at these rules, the harder my life became. Eventually, I was treated like I was toxic, like I was the problem standing between my family and contentment. With parental approval, my siblings picked at my appearance. Your teeth stick out. Your toes are dirty and ugly. You have BO. And my favorite: Brad, your shit stinks worse than anybody else's on the planet.

And, yes, I acknowledge that, on one level, this sounds like standard-fare sibling teasing. But there was a cruelty to it. "Busting on Brad" was never followed with a wink and a hug, let alone an "Aw, but we love you anyway."

The teasing took a toll on my young psyche. If my shit was the smelliest on the planet, then I, my entire being, must be disgusting. I worried that other people saw me as disgusting, too. I tried to shrug it off, but, honestly, it took a toll. Eventually, I became who they told me I was. I wore drab, wrinkled clothing so that my exterior matched how I felt inside. It's no wonder that during my first visit to a psychiatrist I accepted his diagnosis of bipolar disorder without a blink. Hell, being called mentally ill felt far better than being labeled disgusting.

As a kid and a young adult, I was in constant conflict about and with my family, and yet I needed them—of course. This dance, this push-pull, of wanting to be part of something while feeling totally alien from it ran through my nervous system like poison. In the quiet privacy of my room, I pored over the Bible, prayed earnestly to Jesus, and, one weird night, stared in the bathroom mirror at my pubescent scruff and wondered if I *was* Jesus.

As these painful memories rose inside me, I stopped walking and took a sip of water. I felt both sleepy and anxious at the same time. I wanted to stop, to dissociate, to collapse onto my couch back in Santa Fe. I craved the numbness of the drugs. I longed to disappear. I craved a lorazepam. I craved a Dexedrine, a beer, a one-night stand.

After the existential slap in the face that was Paul's death, I'd started tapering off the strongest, most numbing of the drugs. And as the drugs left my system, I experienced positive effects. I felt more aware. More awake. The colors of leaves on the trees seemed brighter. When I listened to music, the textures and subtleties of the sounds sounded richer, too. I was waking up. I'd left the lorazepam at home in Santa Fe. I was aware that I had Dexedrine in my pocket, but I couldn't jack myself up on amphetamines to escape anymore.

Breathe, Brad. You've got this.

As wonderful as it was to be gaining more awareness, more perspective, there were downsides to not being so heavily medicated. My nervous system felt ragged, like there was gravel lodged in every cell of it. I'd felt like this in my teens and early twenties before I began taking meds. I was also dealing with intense withdrawal symptoms. Nighttime was worst: I would lie down and fall asleep, but as soon as I did, my legs would begin to jerk on their own and I'd wake up with a start. It felt like there were bugs or tiny worms in my thighs and calves. The urge to move them was strong, so I moved to relieve the antsy itch, but it provided only temporary relief. The moment I was still, the urge to move them would start to build again. Restless legs sounds like a minor nuisance, but it's excruciating. Over weeks and months of sleepless nights, I was miserable. I was about to push into that purely emotional space created by exhaustion.

Worse still, I was having episodes of sleep paralysis. I would dream of being deep underwater and unable to breathe or move my limbs. I seemed to be half awake and half asleep. I knew that I couldn't breathe, and yet I couldn't draw a breath. I would try to scream. But no scream would come out of my mouth. I would try harder and harder. Eventually, the muted cries would wake me up, and I would lie there panting, soaked in sweat.

I was doing better, but I certainly wasn't well.

The trail crossed farms and wound through Arab villages. Barking dogs. Ancient trees. By 3 p.m., I was walking into the town of Cana, past T-shirt shops and stands selling tchotchkes. I went inside a white church and sat in a pew and knelt. I wanted to pray, but I didn't know what to say. It felt strange showing up in Jesus's house after all these years and asking for something. I set my head in my hands and cried a bit—from the exhaustion, from coming off my meds, from not knowing what the fuck I was looking for or how I would feel or react if I found it. And then I got up, headed out of the church and back into the sunlight, and began walking again. I dug within and found something positive to focus on: I had a beautiful girlfriend. I would write a great article for the *New York Times*. I put my head down and thought about Jesus.

Over the next three days, I traveled across Galilee. I spent the night in cozy cabins and in a dorm at a kibbutz. I engaged in warm conversations with my hosts about family, cultural differences, and religion. Each morning, I strapped on my backpack and walked.

I walked along the ancient stony road to Damascus. I walked up the Horns of Hattin. I passed the ruins of a synagogue from Jesus's time, and then walked to the cliffs of Arbel, with its pocked caves where more than one rebellious, messianic Jew had hidden out and plotted attacks on Roman troops. I thought about my future. I tried not to berate myself about my fucked-up past.

Next up was the Mount of Beatitudes, where Jesus preached the centerpiece of his radical understanding of morality and spirituality. How a surly, lonely teenager like me managed to find meaning, and maybe himself, in these words, I have no clue. But I did, sprinkled in with the melancholy lyrics of Neil Young and James Taylor.

> *Blessed are the poor in spirit, for theirs is the kingdom of heaven.*
> *Blessed are they who mourn, for they shall be comforted.*
> *Blessed are the meek, for they shall inherit the earth.*
> *Blessed are they who hunger and thirst for righteousness, for they shall be satisfied.*
> *Blessed are the merciful, for they shall obtain mercy.*
> *Blessed are the pure of heart, for they shall see God.*
> *Blessed are the peacemakers, for they shall be called children of God.*
> *Blessed are they who are persecuted for the sake of righteousness, for theirs is the kingdom of heaven.*

This landscape had lived in my teenaged imagination, and I was finally there. I wasn't quite sure what to do with that fact and how to be present to the immensity of it.

After four sweaty, hot, dusty, thoughtful days, the trail ended in Capernaum. It felt good to take off my pack and soak my feet in the Sea of Galilee. I was proud of myself. The pills were still in my pocket, untouched.

———

THE HIKE COMPLETE, I phoned the Fauzi Azar, my hostel in Nazareth, and a driver took me back to where my journey had begun. I grabbed my things from my room, hugged Suraida, the hostel manager I'd befriended, and lifted my backpack onto my shoulders. I walked out the garden gate, passed the orange, hand-painted Jesus Trail sign where I'd started those forty miles, and down a street so narrow I could spread my arms and touch the thousand-year-old stone walls on either side. One final time, I took in the blended sound of Christian church bells and Arabic prayers coming from the mosques. Then I walked away from the Old City and into the modern part of Nazareth, which was entirely different. Instead of Ottoman-era stone buildings with flying arches and ornately painted ceilings, I was back among late capitalism's strip malls with pedicure shops, fast-food falafel joints, and gas stations. I continued walking, faster now, toward my next experience. I found my car where I'd parked it behind the gas station, tossed my pack in the trunk, and five minutes later I was zipping along a two-lane highway through the rural outskirts of Nazareth.

As I drove away from Nazareth, I felt a familiar and very difficult feeling rising from my solar plexus. The feeling had a color: dark, shadowy. It had a bilious flavor: fear. Fear and loneliness. I even feared the feeling of fear. And, well, no matter how hard we want to or try to, we cannot run from ourselves. Sometimes healing is about staying put, staying still, staying in your body. And I had tried as hard as I could on that hike, but I was exhausted and didn't have many tools yet to overcome my instinct to run.

As the feeling intensified, I tried to control it with my breathing pattern. First, I breathed deeply. Then I tried rapid breathing, and when that didn't work—of course—I pressed harder on the gas pedal. I turned up the radio. I grabbed a granola bar and gnawed it out of the package, too eager to fix this feeling to properly unwrap it. I wanted a lorazepam. I needed a lorazepam. And barring that, I knew that if I could create a more stressful, sensory experience for myself, I just might be able to forget about the black, melting terror, like tar, spreading within. If I could find a woman to sleep with, I would feel better. I felt greedy, like a hungry ghost. This was the man I remembered, the man who went on the drugs in the first place. This was the reason I disappeared. And I was in no position to say no to these feelings, these needs and wants, at this moment.

I stopped at a gas station, fueled up, and bought a large coffee and a package of Gummi Bears. Caffeine. Sugar.

I got back into my car and followed Highway 60 toward Jerusalem. The gentle hills of Galilee were behind me now, and the landscape was becoming more industrial and urban. The massive concrete Separation Barrier dividing Israel proper and the Occupied West Bank came into view. I was buzzing now. The adrenaline, caffeine, and sugar, and the question, *What will tonight bring?* fueled a distracting urge that propelled me forward. I wanted to get to Jerusalem. I felt like having a beer in a bar and, with luck, talking to a woman, and after that, who knew? I wanted my fix, and I wanted it NOW.

The only thing on my schedule this week was an appointment on Friday with Dr. Pesach Lichtenberg, a psychiatrist at Jerusalem's Herzog Hospital, a man known as the Messiah Doctor, the world's expert in treating Jerusalem syndrome, a somewhat common temporary mental illness that befalls some visitors to the Holy Land. Sufferers believe they *are* the Messiah. I had been mulling over a book proposal about the phenomenon, along with other similar temporary mental illnesses such as Stendhal syndrome and Stockholm syndrome. My mind drifted as I drove.

Near Shoham, the highway bent eastward toward West Jerusalem. I was excited to see the hills of Jerusalem. I imagined all the Jesus sites there. The Via Dolorosa, the street that Jesus walked, carrying the cross, from Pontius Pilate's prison to Golgotha, the hill where he was crucified. The Garden of Gethsemane, where Jesus made a last-ditch prayer to his Father, asking him to stop the madness and spare his life. The Temple Mount, where Jesus, full of righteous anger, flipped over the tables of the money changers and scolded the religious establishment for its moral tyranny.

The traffic on Highway 60 became a snarl. I saw the Mount of Olives, with its vast graveyard. When I was a kid, I learned that Jesus, at his Second Coming, would appear in the clouds over the Mount of Olives and save humanity's ass. I saw the golden Dome of the Rock and the gray-black Al-Aqsa Mosque. And, of course, the ancient limestone walls of the Old City. I could feel the hot shower on my back. I could taste the cold beer at the hostel watering hole. I could see the beautiful woman I hoped to meet there. And tomorrow, I could be walking in the Old City and connecting with the story of Jesus's last week alive and his crucifixion on Golgotha.

Then I saw a sign for Qalandia. I knew that word. Anybody who follows the Israel/Palestine conflict knows that the border crossing is the most famous and heavily guarded public checkpoint in the world. If you are near Jerusalem and you are a non-Israeli—a Palestinian or a foreigner—and you want to cross from Israel to Palestine or from Palestine to Israel, Qalandia is where you do it. I steered onto the exit ramp.

I saw the line of cars waiting to pass into Palestine and drove toward it. I eased my car in behind a rusty white Toyota and put it into park. I turned up the volume on the music pouring out of the tinny dashboard speakers: U2's "I Still Haven't Found What I'm Looking For," with its ringing guitar chords and earnest, grandiose lyrics. I rolled down the window and stuck my head out, trying to assess how long it would take me to get to the front of the line.

There were ten cars up ahead. It was taking the armed guards about five minutes to interview each driver and check for bombs, so I calculated it might take an hour. Could I sit still that long? Would my wait be rewarded with some adventure?

I was trying to heal, but there I was, making the same mistakes, trying to find the road out instead of the road in. It would be many more years before I learned to stop this toxic thrill seeking and vicarious trauma consumption. At the time, I didn't understand how my nervous system had been wired in childhood for thrill seeking. Weirdly, danger had a soothing feeling because it was familiar, and I was hit with it now like a punch in the face. I wanted more. I wanted to see more blown-out buildings, more military traffic stops, more skirting around rioters, more olive groves burning to the ground.

I checked my watch. *Maybe this is a dumb idea. I'm supposed to check in to my hotel in Jerusalem in a few hours. Can I push the interview to later in the week? Can I cancel my reservation if this Palestine trip turns into something exciting?* I felt alive again, maybe for the first time in six or seven years. Is that how long it had been since I started taking that deadly cocktail of antipsychotic medications in addition to antidepressants, mood stabilizers, sedatives, stimulants, sleeping pills, and more? I was working again. I was doing what I loved. It felt so good to be writing again—and for the *New York Times*, no less. This was what I was good at, being a travel journalist. I knew I should be going back to Jerusalem tonight, but the lure of adventure, of following my nose—and not just for a story, not just for a job, was pushing me forward like a strong hand on my back.

I wiped sweat from my brow with the red bandana that I'd carried in my pocket throughout the week. I stuck my head out the window again to calculate my wait time. *Shit.* Only one car had made it through since I last checked. This was going to take longer than I thought. I breathed. I settled into my seat. I played with the air conditioner dials, trying to get the snow to stop blowing out my vents.

Soon I was gone again, dissociating, out of my body and out of this place and time. The sniper towers blurred from the foreground, and I was back at Sylvie's house. Though my body was sitting in a car at Qalandia, my mind and entire nervous system was simultaneously entering a vivid PTSD flashback. I was in Santa Fe, on the carpet next to Paul's blue, cold body. I started to cry. My mouth felt as wide open as Munch's scream. And the tears wouldn't stop. I covered my mouth with my arm. *Men don't cry*, I told myself, *What if someone sees you?* But the weeping continued, and I was breathing fast and hard. And then, as quickly as the tears had flowed, they stopped. I felt my body relax, and I sat back in my seat. The breathing slowed.

My eyes refocused on my immediate surroundings. I looked around at the wasteland of desert, the concrete sniper towers, and the border guards in their bulletproof vests. This was one of the most dangerous places in the world. The Israeli army ruled it with absolute and deadly force. Palestinians expressed their rage there in rock-throwing protests. When the two collided, there were shootings, fires, lynchings, deaths.

I tried to distract myself with wondering what Andrea was up to. She and I had been together for a year. She was beautiful and kind and deep. It was on again, off again. I couldn't feel my deepest feelings, and I didn't know whether what I felt for her was love or lust. And I thought about my mother, back in Kansas in so much pain, suffering from stage 4 melanoma that had spread to her liver and bones. My body ached for her presence. I didn't see her as much as I wanted to. She was still with my father, and visits home tended not to go very well.

The line was moving now. I was the fifth car. *Time to focus: What are you going to say to the heavily armed soldier if he asks you what you intend to do in Palestine? Don't say you're a journalist. That will only lead to more questions. What am I planning to do in Palestine? What should I tell him?*

"What am I doing here? Well, sir, I was a Jesus freak when I was a kid, a fundamentalist Christian, you know, the kind that America is full of. They read the Bible literally. They think Jesus is going to show up in the sky over Jerusalem in a few years, maybe next year, and start his eternal earthly reign. But before that, there's going to be World War III on your soil. We say cute rhyming prayers and talk about Jesus as if he's in the room with us right now. Our friend, and our Lord and Savior. You've probably seen the baseball-playing version of us: when we hit a home run, we point to the sky to the Big Man Upstairs! Well, I'm not that now. I'm basically a drug addict. I spent the past five years taking twelve prescription drugs, twenty-three pills per day, even antipsychotics, espe-cially uppers and downers and sleeping pills and mood stabilizers . . . and even a drug to curb my appetite because the antipsychotic made me eat endless bowls of cereal. And, well, I'm trying to find myself. And I'm basically broke. At night I have bad cravings for the drugs I just stopped taking, my legs wiggle, and I can't stay asleep more than a few hours. And well, I thought that I might do a little personal research into Jesus. I'm wondering if I could be, um, a Christian again."

Nope, that won't work. That is way too much information. You sound like a manic depressive on the upswing. Slow the fuck down, Brad. Say all that and he'll think you really are crazy. Am I crazy?

I rehearsed another speech:

"Well, sir, I just finished reporting a travel article for the *New York Times* about the Jesus Trail. I hiked the forty miles between Nazareth, childhood home of Jesus, and the Sea of Galilee, where he found his dis-ciples and began his ministry. And, well, I was driving back to Jerusalem, and I saw the turn off for Palestine, and I want to take a look, see?"

Well, that's honest, and honesty is usually the best policy, but that's too much information still. Slow. The fuck. Down. What does he really need to know?

This came out next, and this time I practiced out loud as I moved one more car's length closer to the guards.

"I'm a tourist. I want to see the River Jordan and other sites."

Then I remembered something I'd heard at the hostel. "They'll want to know your religion. They don't want Israeli Jews going there. They don't want them to see what's up. They don't want to know what kind of Christian you are. They don't want to know you're a lapsed Christian. They only know Catholic and Orthodox and that's it. Just say, I'm Christian."

Finally, I settled on the short-and-sweet-approach: "I'm a tourist. I'm Christian."

I took a deep breath and then another, but it didn't settle my ner-vous system. Bono was still crooning. I started matching my breath to the beat of the song, just to distract myself. I didn't even know what I was so ramped up about. I was hot, not from the temperature, but from all the nervous energy I was generating. It was not anxiety, exactly, but maybe those close cousins: adrenaline, anxiety, joy, terror. Pretty much every emotion that a caveman might have felt when he spotted a woolly mammoth and knew it was game time.

I wished I had a lorazepam, or a propanolol, which although not as good as a lorazepam, would keep my heart from pounding this hole in my chest. But no. I was committed to not taking it anymore. I left most of the good stuff back in New Mexico. I could see the bottles now, jammed haphazardly into my medicine cabinet.

Breathe, Brad. Breathe, Brad.

I tried breathing exercises I learned in yoga class. I thought about the mindfulness class my therapist told me to take. But I couldn't calm myself enough in class to learn anything.

I started to laugh. Nobody who looked at my resume or read my adventure stories would know how fucked up inside I'd felt for most of my life. I was full of sweeping emotions now. I felt like a teenager. Maybe the teenager I couldn't be because I was depressed. Maybe the teenager I was before I started taking all the pills. Maybe all the emotions that were coming through me included every emotion I was supposed to feel but couldn't back then. All of them at once—here they were. They weren't allowed, and as I grew up, I didn't allow myself to feel them. And they were big, and they scared me. I didn't know what to do with them.

If I had known what to do with them, I wouldn't be here, at the most dangerous border crossing in the world. I would have been home golfing with my CEO buddies, looking up from my putter to tell them which colleges my kids were going to. Or taking my wife to a fancy dinner with the best bottle of wine the restaurant had to offer.

But I was where I was. And I was at a personal threshold, as well. I couldn't go back. But I didn't know how to go forward. I had no itinerary. I lacked a letter from a company or government explaining who I was and why I was there. I knew nobody. Not a soul, not my family, friends, or significant other at the time had a clue where I was or where I was going. Hell, I didn't know.

I was now second in line.

I was pleased with my story about being a Christian tourist, but suddenly I was unhappy with the temperature—nearly as hot inside my car as outside. I reached to turn up the air conditioner. As soon as my finger touched the lever, the dashboard let out a groan, then a burp, then a hiss. The vents blew snowflakes for thirty seconds. And then, nothing. I was sweating through my clothes. I rolled down the window and stuck out my elbow.

And now it was my turn. The soldier sidled up to my car window. I handed him my passport. He flipped through the pages, glancing up occasionally to look me in the eye. He asked me why I was there. I told him my Christian tourist story. I embellished it by adding that I'd long dreamed of being baptized in the River Jordan. I wanted to see where the devil tempted Jesus. The soldier laughed. I laughed. He asked me to pop the trunk. I followed orders. He looked inside, and then slammed the trunk shut. He handed me back my passport and motioned with his gun muzzle for me to pass through.

It was over.

At first, I drove slowly, glancing down side streets at Palestinian men in T-shirts selling bottled water, women in headscarves carrying babies, toddlers toddling. I glanced up at the concrete towers, trying to peer through the slots where the snipers sat, just waiting to blast a third eye through the skulls of anybody who did anything out of the ordinary.

I hit the gas and the car picked up speed through Qalandia's bombed-out neighborhoods. Soon the buildings were farther apart. The city gave way to suburbs and eventually to lonely, white desert that sloped steeply down, down, down toward Jericho and the Dead Sea, the lowest, hottest place on earth. *I could use a short swim in the River Jordan*, I thought. *Or, maybe, a baptism.*

thirteen

WASHED CLEAN

WHEN I WAS A KID, OUR HOUSE FLOODED. TWICE. DURING heavy summer rains, water from the creek in our front yard flooded the basement and then the first floor, ruining almost everything we owned. Soggy couches, mud-encrusted carpets, and moldy mattresses filled our manicured front lawn. It felt like weeks that my family spent our days breathing moldy air and sitting on the floor, surrounded by buzzing high-speed fans and gurgling dehumidifiers hammering at floor tiles till they cracked and came up. Everything was mold coated and had to be removed. A few years later, when I was in high school, I was home alone for what was almost a third flood. My parents were out of town when it rained hard for two solid days. On the third day, the creek began creeping slowly toward the house. I felt sick to my stomach as it rose above the front step and lapped at the front door. I was planning my escape through waist-high water when the rains miraculously stopped, and the creek receded.

So I know a few things about how we humans deal with an impending, slow-arriving disaster. When the water first begins to rise, we tell ourselves it's not going to happen. We are firm in our disbelief. Thirty minutes later, as the water rises higher, we tell ourselves it will stop. When the water is a foot away from the front door, we think about leaving, but we wait. We deny. We bargain. We hope. Maybe we pray. Only as the water crosses the threshold and begins to consume our furniture do we decide that now is the time to leave. But the water is now so high that we must wade or even swim to safety.

Deciding to be honest with ourselves during hard times is like watching floodwaters rise. We don't face ourselves when we should, but we wait, deny, bargain, hope. By the time we've run through these feeling states, the only remaining option is to act; if we don't, we will be subsumed in our own psychic floods, forced to swim through the muddy water of our minds, desperate for safe shores. We will flail.

As I drove across the golden moonscape that is the Judean Desert, with its wide-lens views of the barren Judean Hills, resembling massive breaching whales, the water of my life was lapping at my door. Having waited too long for a calm and sensible self-rescue, I was scrambling desperately for high ground. Every time I blinked, I saw Paul's dead body lying on the hallway carpet, then my own. *Blink.* Paul. *Blink.* Brad. I couldn't touch the memory of our last conversation, when Paul told me, in so many words, that he planned to end his own life. I couldn't face the seven years I'd just wasted in a miserable, drugged-out haze. That floodwater had filled the basement, and I was terrified to open the door and look down into that watery darkness. It was time to swim to safety. I needed hope. I couldn't say exactly how traveling across Palestine, how following in Jesus's footsteps, how baptizing myself was going to lead to my healing. I just knew that this was what I needed to do. Some deeper part of my psyche — my soul? — was guiding me. Perhaps it was steering the car. I thought of Gene Savoy's words: "If you find a road, take it. A road goes someplace." Was my road out there, somewhere in this moonscape?

At the same time, I did feel ready to get real with myself. I knew I had to make corrections in how I was moving through the world, but I didn't know how. I was confused about my life, particularly my experience with my own family. As I drove, that feeling of being an orphan returned. Why, I wondered. Where did this deep-seated feeling of being outside my family, even outside own life, originate? I racked my brain. But my thoughts swirled. And so I came back to the feeling inside. The feeling, deep, profound loneliness, felt truer than any thought I had. In one corner of my psyche, there was desert that was as stark and empty as the hot, red desert I was driving through. I sat with this feeling, and soon memories from childhood and adulthood swirled around in my head. As a child and after I grew up, my outspokenness about my family's issues made me their enemy. Nobody wanted to hear it. Slowly, I was pushed out and treated like a pariah. After my divorce from Di, I was no longer invited on extended-family vacations, which I learned about from social media. When I did return home for an occasional holiday visit, I faced a family that seemed to see me and my desire for openness and honesty as "the problem." I had been in weekly therapy since I was twenty-five, and I'd read countless self-help books about how to heal my codependency and other effects of growing up with my dysfunctional family. But the one thing I didn't learn—or I was in denial about—was just how reluctant dysfunctional families can be to look at themselves. And how in denial I was about my family. I get it now. Most people don't desire radical honesty. But that more naive Brad who came home at Thanksgiving or Christmas hoping for a different family experience couldn't fathom that they didn't want to talk about feelings or relationships, let alone discuss a path to healing ourselves. And although my father had learned to drink less, he still drank, and, to my experience, he never did a thing to face his own emotional issues or to repair the damage he'd done to our family. Meanwhile, my older brother, David, and his wife, Lisa, both successful attorneys and businesspeople, had ironically embraced drinking as a hobby. They loved talking about their growing wine collection, schmoozing with the sommeliers, and making a pageant of their selections at restaurants. I didn't know a lot about Lisa's family except that her younger sister, the black sheep of their family, had struggled with various addictions and died by suicide before age forty. Lisa rarely spoke about her, and I wondered if they had been close. At holiday dinners, I sat at the table, sipping my sparkling water and listening to everybody blather on about recent changes in local zoning ordinances, the new furniture in the clubhouse at the country club, and other trivial things I didn't know or care about, feeling unseen, frustrated, and angry at the lack of emotional intimacy. "Anybody read a book they liked recently?" I'd blurt out, with an edge to my voice. By dessert, we had all removed our gloves. Insults flew freely and my mother cried.

And yet I knew I couldn't heal all by myself. I needed community— even advice, maybe fatherly advice. But there was nobody I trusted. Obviously, turning to my father wasn't an option. Likewise, David had never seemed interested in being a resource, let alone a friend, to me. After college, he rarely stayed in touch. After we both began our careers, he seldom answered my texts, emails, or calls. I understood that he was busy, but I also seemed to trigger something in him that didn't allow him to show up. Though he was highly successful in business, and he and his wife had won a half-million dollars in the Kansas Lottery, I wondered if he felt threatened by my version of success, my experiences as an adventure writer, my travels, and my connections. He and his family stopped visiting Santa Fe, which had been their favorite place in the world before I moved there. When I called to tell him about my contract with *George* and my note from John F. Kennedy Jr., his voice dropped, and he seemed annoyed. When the extended family got together at holidays, he and Lisa became visibly irritated when I shared stories about my travels. Later, after I stopped writing for publication and my confidence receded behind the fog of drugs, they laughed and rolled their eyes when I said anything about my successful travel-writing career. When Di and I were married, she often walked away from these dinners scratching her head and asking, "Why do they think you haven't been successful? I don't get it." Years later, after our divorce, she occasionally received phone calls from my father and brother on her birthday and holidays, and she confided in me that they still talked about me that way. "It's like they are talking about somebody else."

I now understand the family dynamic better. Or I think I do. As I disappeared into the fog, my family's narrative about me had to shift. They needed to see me as a Walter Mitty, the ordinary guy who fantasized constantly about a more adventurous life than the one he actually lived.

When those Dos Equis beer commercials featuring the Most Interesting Man in the World appeared on television, they laughed and said *that's you, Brad*. (They once persuaded me to pose for a photograph in front of an inflatable Dos Equis bottle. I acquiesced, trying to see it as harmless fun, but it wasn't. It was pure self-betrayal, and it felt terrible.) Like the Most Interesting Man in the World, I was a raging narcissist, a ridiculous liar, and my years of success as an editor, adventure travel writer, columnist, and author of a collection of my nature writings by a major publisher was a figment of my imagination.

This narrative, as hurtful as it was, later became an essential piece of information in my reaching an understanding about what had happened to me: to my life, my spirit, my sense of self. It also highlighted the denial, the dysfunction, the extreme masculine power struggle, and perhaps the toxic narcissism that formed our familial paradigm. Later still, after Donald Trump became president, I found more insight. Trump and his supporters referred to actual facts as "fake news," which was exactly the way I felt my family had treated the facts of my life and, essentially, who I was as a person, as a man: in their eyes, I was a fake. Dr. Frank Yeomans, a professor of psychiatry at Cornell University and a leading expert on personality disorders, explains narcissism as a "defense against reality." He calls it a form of psychosis. A narcissist constantly, and unconsciously, tells himself untrue stories about his life and others' to protect his ego from facts that would be too painful to acknowledge. Whatever was going on with my family, I appeared to have become fake news to them. My stories became fake. I was fake. They seemed to cast me as the family narcissist to avoid looking at their own lives, their own patterns of behavior. Perhaps I did tell too many stories about my travels to impress them or win their love. Maybe I was obnoxious. But I definitely was a successful travel editor and writer for fifteen years.

And yet, looking back on this time, I can see that I was causing myself more suffering by not accepting the reality of this family tragedy. Perhaps they wished they had a different son—and I wished I had a different family. I couldn't yet accept this about them—about me—and save myself from the toxicity by walking away. Of course, I couldn't. Years later, I learned in therapy that "trauma bonds" between people are more difficult to break than loving bonds. The reason: people will idolize the very people who hurt them. It's similar to the way Stockholm Syndrome works.

By the time I arrived in Palestine, I was struggling to regain my own story. I had been willing to abandon myself, my own truth, and the memories of the things I had accomplished. I had believed others' version of me more than I trusted my own. Now, in this holy place, I wondered, What was the true story about my life? I honestly didn't know. Coming here to walk in Jesus's footsteps was my way of seeking a new model, a different paradigm, a solid story to lean on. Jesus was the vital figure from my youth. He seemed to be the ideal man. When you take away the religious aspects of the story, that's the essence of who he was in the world. He was accepting, generous, kind, and sought justice for all. He was someone that we imperfect humans, driven by impulses and fragilities beyond our control, could strive to emulate. Jesus was strong, compassionate, merciful, outspoken, and he wasn't a pushover in the face of powerful men and social organizations. He spoke his mind, and he faced the ultimate consequences. Who wouldn't want to be like Jesus?

With all of this in my mind and heart, I drove across the Judean Desert. Could this weird journey through history, sacred religious scriptures, and my own past show me anything useful about how to rebuild my life? I had to find out.

I saw the turnoff for the baptismal site at Qasr el Yahud on the western bank of the Jordan River, slowed down, exited the highway, and pulled into the parking area.

I was mesmerized—not by the meaning I believed I was about to experience but by the red sign posted on the barbed-wire fence to my right: "Danger Mines!" Beyond the sign and fence was what you'd expect a minefield to look like: acres upon acres of dirt built up into little gopher-like mounds. After the 1967 war, when Israel captured the West Bank from Jordan, the army placed four thousand explosive devices in the ground to prevent anyone from taking back the land.

Qasr el Yahud was also the site of significant Old Testament events; this bend in the river was the place where, according to Jewish tradition, the Israelites crossed the Jordan and entered the Promised Land for the first time. It's also the place where tradition says the prophet Ezekiel ascended to heaven.

Wow, I thought as I stepped out of the car and onto the hot pavement. *A minefield next to the site where Jesus experienced his spiritual rebirth and where the Jewish people first entered the Promised Land?* It felt to me like a literal minefield of mixed messages.

I walked toward the cluster of palm trees that lined the river. The pavement stuck to my flip-flops like chewing gum. The minefield disturbed me deeply, even if it was on the other side of a fence and I could easily steer clear. That wasn't possible with another frightening thing, parked under a palm tree: a massive bus with a sign in the windshield indicating its passengers were members of a church in Dallas, Texas.

I couldn't help but smile.

The church folks from Texas mobbed the visitor's center, though I admit they were less scary in person than in theory. It was a quiet, sweet, multiracial group of men and women huddled on the wood steps, all descending to the water. I smiled and waved to an older woman who looked so ecstatic—as if she'd just won the Texas Powerball. I kept moving to the far side of the wood steps to sit and take in the scene.

That's when I noticed John the Baptist standing chest-high in the middle of the narrow, easy-moving river. A heavyset, blond man with a matching goatee, I figured he was the pastor, playing the part for the group. He wore a white robe that exposed his hairy chest. It wasn't a camel-hair shirt like the original John the Baptist was said to have worn, but this modern John fit the part perfectly. His face beamed. He looked utterly rapturous. I wondered briefly if this crew was on ecstasy.

A middle-aged woman with a boyish haircut stood in the water next to modern John. His hand rested on the crown of her head, and he was reciting a prayer that I couldn't make out. She was crying joyfully and appeared to be in a state of blissful spiritual overwhelm. Then he looked her in the eye and seemed to ask, *Are you ready?* She nodded. He placed one hand on her shoulder and the other against her lower back. He pushed her back gently until she disappeared under the water for a full second. After helping her resurface, he cupped his hands and poured three successive palmfuls of water over her head. By now, she was weeping loudly. He hugged her, and then, with one hand resting on his own heart, he gestured with the other hand that it was time for her to wade back to shore. She climbed out of the water and back onto the wood steps, at which time another church member—an elderly man with short gray hair, wearing horn-rimmed glasses—stepped gingerly off the riser into the water and waded out. I watched as the pastor repeated the ritual with this man and then again with two other church members. Given that the scene involved Americans, the group baptism could have felt showbiz, but I was pleasantly surprised by how touching and peaceful it was.

The baptisms continued, but I had seen enough. I moved to a dry patch of grass far enough away that I couldn't hear the others. I reflected on the story of Jesus's baptism, which I still knew quite well a good thirty years after I'd studied it so intently.

Sometime around his thirtieth birthday, Jesus left his home in Nazareth and traveled on foot roughly a hundred miles to Jerusalem. It was there he learned about John the Baptist, a renegade, wild man figure who had made a reputation for himself performing a new type of spiritual cleansing in the Jordan River, an adaption of the longstanding Jewish ritual of frequently purifying oneself by bathing in blessed water. John also taught that repentance and bathing in spiritual waters were the paths to the forgiveness of sins. Jesus walked east, toward the Jordan, to receive this purification. Water, particularly moving water, has long been a symbol of spiritual cleansing and of spirit itself. The Gospel of Mark refers to the promise made in the book of Isaiah: that when the Messiah appeared, God would send somebody "before him." Christians believe that John the Baptist was that person.

When Jesus arrived, John recognized his greatness and said that Jesus should be baptizing him, not the other way around. But Jesus insisted.

John doused him and blessed him. Then, according to the biblical narrative, the heavens opened, and the Holy Spirit descended "like a dove," landing on Jesus. It was then that Jesus fully embraced his identity as the Son of God. Things didn't go so well for John: the Jewish priestly caste saw him as a threat and eventually had him beheaded. His severed head was delivered on a platter to the Roman ruler, Herod Antipas, in 30 CE.

Palestine, as the region was called, was at that time controlled by two layers of authority: a religious layer—Jewish leaders of the Temple—and a civic layer—Rome. The Roman prefect during the time of Jesus, Pontius Pilate, held the political power, but he worked closely with the Temple priests to maintain order. He wasn't stupid. He knew he needed the priests to keep the masses happy and, in some cases, at bay.

The Christian analysis is that the Jewish religion had become highly ritualized and commercialized at the time—not unlike the commercialization of Catholic practices during medieval times. To be forgiven of sins, one had to make frequent visits to the Temple, buy animals for sacrifice, and then pay a priest to perform that sacrifice on your behalf inside the Temple. Such activities would appease God and keep the crops growing and the sun rising on schedule. This worked for some people. But if you couldn't afford these rituals or you envisioned spiritual life differently than what you'd been taught to believe, you might have been drawn to John the Baptist or the Zealots, men seen as liberators of the Jews from the demands of both the traditional priests and Roman leadership. It's not hard to picture being on the lookout for the Messiah the Scriptures told you was on the way. You might have mourned John the Baptist's murder, and you might have been willing to see this Jesus person as somebody of substance. These stories are ancient, but it's maybe not that hard to picture them happening today, too—wanting your religion to be revolutionized by someone genuine and grounded, someone who was directly empowering your life, your money, and your spirituality.

Now, thousands of years later, I was sitting on a patch of grass at the location where Jesus received his first hit of divine inspiration and launched his world-changing spiritual crusade. I had felt a pressure in my body, a necessity, to see this place with my own eyes and to experience it in my own body. I hoped it would help me see something new about myself or remember something—I wasn't sure which. Could I find divine inspiration here, too, like Jesus had? I was no savior, I knew that. Far from it. I lacked a job, let alone purpose. But I was still a seeker, and I came here seeking something. I'd been housebound for so many years, slowly trying to rid myself of all that ambition that had driven me to be an adventure writer.

The word "ego" is confusing. In Eastern spirituality, it has a negative connotation: it is the selfish part of us that gets in the way of achieving enlightenment. The work of our lives is to transcend the ego, to connect with the inner observer that already sees that our personality, our stories, are not who we really are. When we connect with the self, we see our soul. And because our soul is connected to the souls of everybody and the soul of the world, we connect with God. In other words, we can meditate our way to God consciousness. But the ego has a far different meaning—and purpose—in the Western psychological tradition. Ego is how we relate to the world. We need a sufficiently strong ego to earn a living, negotiate relationships, live with meaning and purpose, and so on. Many people who show up in treatment for mental illnesses have an undeveloped or fractured ego. Our ego is the part of our minds that must face the bumps and curves of the real world. You don't want an *overdeveloped* ego—which is an imperfect definition of narcissism, when all you care about is yourself and you mow over anyone who gets in the way of your desires or end goal. This type occupies the halls of politics, the executive suites of Wall Street, and sidles up to bars around the country every night. But you also don't want an undeveloped ego. After my collapse, all that high-test ambition drained away, revealing the truth that ambition and grandiosity overcompensating for my toxic shame and unworthiness had functioned as my ego. I felt as though I didn't have a solid center, a sense of being grounded in who I was at my core. What was left of me when you took away the career, the relationship, the family, the pills? I felt as murky as the muddy Jordan.

I wouldn't have described it like this in 2012, but I now see that I needed to build a healthy ego, which had been squashed during my childhood years. In 2012 I couldn't articulate this as the problem, so I had no idea how to fix it. I needed to rebuild myself, but there was no map because I was unsure of the starting point—me. I knew I did *not* want to become just another asshole American man, overly focused on achievement, money, acquisition, competition, woefully disconnected from his feelings apart from anger. I had played that game, and I wasn't interested in rebuilding my life only to fall back into the same traps that led me to my breakdown in the first place. I wasn't about to return to society to work my ass off to buy a monster pickup truck or remodel my basement into an exquisite entertainment center. I didn't want any part of the American Dream, but I had no dream with which to replace it. And now, I simply didn't feel a newly restored faith in Jesus that might inspire a clear path forward, which is something I half wished this trip to the birthplace of Christianity might inspire.

The only thing I knew—a small, quiet part of my gut knew—was that spirituality might play a significant part in what I needed to structure a life that mattered to me. Every spiritual path I was aware of asked the same thing of its followers: humility. I had learned in my childhood Bible study classes that if we want to be transformed, we must begin with humility about where we are starting from. And I was ready for that. I didn't have any reason not to be humble. I had very little going for me. Everything I'd done to try to feel better had failed: sex, travel, drugs, self-help books, relationships, psychiatrists, life coaches. How was it that I was forty-six years old and felt no better than I did the day I left my home in Kansas for college, no better than during those sleepless nights when I read the Bible after walking my dad to bed?

Full of self-pity, I tossed a small stick into the river and watched it float southward toward the Dead Sea. I knew it would never arrive there.

I'd read that the Jordan River was drying up; a few miles from here, this gently flowing stream slowed to a trickle and eventually became sandy riverbed. I felt like doing a disappearing act myself.

I had hoped I would feel differently here; I thought I might have a Saul-like lightning bolt moment and become my version of Paul. I'd hoped to feel inspired, invigorated, ready to take on the next chapter of my life. Even if I didn't believe in Jesus Christ, I'd hoped that if I sat by the Jordan, maybe I might feel the Holy Spirit entering me—or some kind of spirit. Becoming a Jesus freak again would have been inconvenient, but it would at least give me a path forward with clear benchmarks of my progress. I'd hoped that maybe here I would feel Jesus's famous love as described in the lyrics to the song: "Jesus loves me, this I know." I'd hoped for so much, but writing this now, I understand that hope is not a useful strategy for self-transformation. As we try to morph and change, we must embrace a certain amount of optimism that we can get to the other side, that our lives can get better, that the shit will shift. Without optimism, it can be difficult to do the hard work of going to yoga classes, meditating regularly, showing up and being present at therapy sessions. But hope—wishing things would get better or praying that our lives or the world were different—is useless. On that day, I was still leaning too heavily on hope.

As the stick I'd tossed disappeared around the bend, I noticed that it was quiet and I was alone. The Texans had left the river and were back at the bus waiting to board. I felt a little prickle of heat move through me. A small sense of excitement about being alone in this popular sacred spot pushed through the lethargic, deadening weight of my hopeless thoughts.

I don't think I consciously decided to do what I did next.

I looked around once more to make sure I was truly alone. I removed my sandals and shirt. I pulled my shorts up around my waist and removed my sunglasses, setting them on top of my sandals. Then I turned my gaze to the center of the river to the deep spot where the contemporary John the Baptist had just been standing, blessing his flock with gentle dunks in the water. I stepped off the wooden stairs and into the river. Ankle high. I took another step. Knee high. And another. Thigh high. And then waist high. Until I was standing in the middle of the Jordan River up to my chest. The water was tepid and murky, unlike the fresh, cool streams from Colorado near my home. But at this moment, that didn't matter. It felt deeply cleansing, even life preserving. Unlike the floodwaters of my youth, I welcomed the murkiness, too, as the water rose against my torso. Instead of fleeing these waters, I wanted the stream to fill me up, replace my own blood.

I looked up toward Jerusalem. I was still alone, which felt like a small miracle in and of itself. I inhaled. I exhaled. And then again. I felt nervous. But why? What was the point of any of this? And then I took a breath so big I thought I might float into space. I bent my knees and let my feet off the river floor. My head dropped under water. I stayed there. I paused, my eyes squeezed tight against the muddy water, my breath slowly exiting my nose.

Do I have to come up? My mind drifted back to that May afternoon on the White River in Arkansas. I felt the hard, rough log against my skinny-kid torso. I felt the broken branches dig into my skin. I felt the upriver current pushing me hard into the log. I felt the downriver current pulling at my spindly limbs. In that weird way in which so much can happen in an instant, I found myself wondering how big a container I'd need to hold all the pills I'd stuffed down my throat over the years with the hope that they would save me, make me different, make me whole. A pickup? A dump truck? A garbage truck? Then I imagined the drugs, which still were in my bloodstream at a disturbingly high level, being washed away downriver. I imagined my sins washed away. All of them.

I found my footing on the sand and stood up. As my head emerged from the water, I felt a wellspring of emotion rise from my belly through my chest, neck, and jaw, and then tears burst from my eyes. I wept loudly.

Jesus Christ, where the hell are you? Where's the love? Where's the kindness? Where's the fucking grace?

As I stepped out of the river, a new feeling pulsated through my body, warm and full. It moved like energy but felt solid at the same time. Strong, too. This feeling filled my legs and then my torso. It felt like hot, liquid steel was being poured into the mold of my body. It felt like power but without the edge. It was directed at nobody. It simply was. I tried to make sense of it with words: it felt like survival. I was here. Still here. I was alive, in this body, in this river, in this moment, right now. I had made it through the darkest days when I was convinced that I might not make it through the night, too confused about who I was, why I felt so alone. At times, I had felt like I was truly dying from the inside.

But I didn't die. And I was not going to. Not now. I was going to find my way back home. Not to Kansas. To me.

Back in my car, the hot vinyl seats seared the skin on my legs. My clothes felt swampy after the river dunk. I started up the car and drove slowly past the "Danger Mines!" sign. How enthusiastic, this sign, and how deeply sad. I rolled past the barbed wire and mounds of dirt and rejoined the highway.

I was confused about what I'd just done, and yet I felt hopeful that it had been more than a silly recreation or a passing moment of folly or fear. I desperately wanted it to mean something more, to mark what I craved to be true: No more chaos. No more shame. No more suffering. Admittedly, I was a little too hopeful. I was again placing my hopes on something external that might save me, contain me, heal me. But this time that thing wasn't a pill or a woman or a promotion or a hot story or an accolade. That, I knew, *I believed,* was a start, and a deeply important one. The trance of my life—the shame, the avoidance, the escapism, the cocktail of medication—hadn't been washed away. I was still in that trance. The difference was that I'd spotted the exit. Now the only question was, How do I open the door?

fourteen

A HIKE WITH SATAN

WEEKS BEFORE MY TRIP, I'D FOUND MY CHILDHOOD BIBLE in my storage unit on a hot Saturday afternoon when I was organizing my things to sell at the Sunday flea market. Since then, I'd been poring over the passages I'd read as a teenager, marked with underlines and barely comprehensible margin notes about how I could live the spirit of the Scriptures in my life. I found a few wise remarks about how I needed to love the obnoxious people in my class, in addition to more than one admonition against masturbation. Jesus didn't say anything about it, as far as I could find, but as I teenager I had a strong sense he wouldn't have wanted me to.

As I drove away from the river en route to Jerusalem, I wanted to stay clean of the drugs. And I knew I would need strength—maybe even Holy Spirit–levels of strength—to continue to reduce dosages once I returned home. I sensed my time in the Jordan wasn't going to solve that one for me completely. As I drove, my thoughts fell back into a familiar groove, working and reworking my childhood, especially my difficult relationship with my father. I rarely experienced attunement or repair with him. Eventually, I stopped trusting him, and I think he responded with ambivalence toward me, sometimes outright dismissal. I've read in books about childhood trauma that a child learns how to trust his own instincts from having a trusting relationships with parents. A child who grows up with a parent who distorts reality through denial and lies will struggle to trust their own judgments of reality, the universe, and even themselves. They will be unable to develop healthy attachments with others. When I spoke up in frustration about how he couldn't see who I was, he accused me of being angry or told me that I was hurting him. And if I didn't speak my mind, if I closed myself in my room and read the Bible to try to comfort myself, I felt the sick feeling of weakness, and right behind that was the equally terrible feeling of having betrayed myself. Either way, I went to bed feeling like everything was my fault. Fault stuck to me like dog shit on my shoe, tracking shame everywhere I went. I felt gutted. I began to distrust him and the rest of my family, too. Eventually, I lived with them, but as an outsider. And this feeling of being an outsider in my own family led me at times to feel so frustrated and alone that I said hurtful things, too. Did they push me out? Or did I slowly, day by day, leave on my own accord? Could both be true?

Jesus Christ! Life is so complicated, I thought as I rummaged around on the car floor for a bottle of water. *At least, Jesus didn't have to deal with psychological thinking. But man, his dad was demanding too. Far more than mine.*

There was no water to be found, so I opened my audiobook app to listen to what came next after Jesus's baptism.

His journey now clear, Jesus departed the Jordan for the "wilderness"— the land around the nearby city of Jericho—where he meditated and fasted for forty days before encountering Satan, who presented him with three temptations. However, by this time, Jesus was on fire spiritually speaking; he was fully tested and ready to begin his ministry. He high-tailed it back to Nazareth, where he began teaching in the synagogues before he was chased out of town by angry locals who accused him of committing blasphemy by suggesting that he was the Son of God.

The air was heating up. I guessed it must be at least 100 degrees. I really needed something to drink. I wondered whether there were 7-Elevens in Palestine when I saw a sign for Jericho and remembered the Old Testament story of the Wall of Jericho, about a prostitute who believed in God and was therefore saved from destruction when it fell. I pulled off the highway, looking for a store that might sell cold drinks, and found myself in a dirt parking lot featuring a camel and a lemonade stand.

At the lemonade stand I ordered two lemonades from the Palestinian owner.

"What's with the camel?" I asked. The camel stood perfectly still except for its mouth; it made weird grimaces and stuck its tongue out. I watched the man squeeze the juice of two lemons into a jar, add water and sugar, and stir.

"For tourists. I give camel rides. You want one?"

"No, thank you. But it's an impressive animal. Can they really go a long time without drinking water?" That was all I could think to ask.

"I don't know," he said. "It's my brother's camel. I run the lemonade stand and offer camel rides to kids."

We chatted about Jericho and the recent tensions between Israel, the United States, and Iran, and he told me about this life in Palestine, which sounded difficult and frightening. He told me about a recent harrowing experience. He was returning to the West Bank from Jordan, and as he came through the border crossing, he was taken to prison for two days and nights. "They treated me like I was a terrorist," he said. "I told them I am not a terrorist. I sell lemonade in a parking lot in Jericho." The man was furious as he retold the story.

His words hurt my heart. I tried to imagine his longing, the longing to feel seen and heard and have a homeland. And, of course, I know that the same longing for home had driven people to Israel as well. Hurt people hurt people. My problems seemed petty in comparison to the complicated, thousand-year-old conflict in the Middle East.

"I'm sorry you went through that," I said. "I don't know what to say. I can't imagine."

"Tell your American friends that we are not all terrorists," he said.

I thanked him for the lemonade and drank it while sitting on the hood of my car.

"You should go to the park and see the famous Wall of Jericho," he suggested.

"Maybe. I'm just coming from Qasr al Yahud. I saw where Jesus was baptized."

"Very nice," he said. "Are you a Christian?"

I wasn't sure how to answer, but I knew it wasn't a simple yes or no. "Not really. I was when I was a kid. But I haven't been one for a very long time." I told him that I was writing an article about the Jesus Trail and that I wanted to see other sights associated with him. Thus, I went to Qasr al Yahud, and I planned to go to Bethlehem.

"Not the Mount of Temptation?"

"What's that?"

"It's right there. That mountain. That's the mountain where Satan tempted Jesus. The gondola takes you to the top. You should see it. There's a monastery and a restaurant up there, too. Very nice."

"I guess I haven't read about the Mount of Temptation yet. Can I just walk up there instead of taking the lift?"

"Of course. But it's hot. The gondola is very nice and fast, too."

"I don't want to take the gondola. But I do want to see where Jesus met Satan."

The man pointed me down a street, explaining that the trail began where the street ended. I thanked him for the lemonade and advice, locked my car, and then I took off down the street until it turned into a trail, headed toward a red cliff face. The rock reminded me of the Organ Mountains in southern New Mexico near Las Cruces. The trail steepened, and I looked up at the tram cars swinging in the hot sun. My breathing grew faster and harder, but I didn't regret taking the hard way. Between the steps at Nazareth and this place, Jesus must have been in good physical shape.

Like so many popular natural places that would ideally be kept wild, the Mount of Temptation is topped off by a restaurant. I wasn't interested. I gazed through the window and saw a waitress rolling silverware into napkins. I scampered down the trail, which followed the side of the steep wall like a goat path. Then I came to a cave with a hand-painted wooden sign leaning against the rock wall: "Meditation Cave." Were we to presume that Jesus meditated in this cave?

The opening was large and welcoming. Inside the smooth limestone walls were cool to the touch, a respite from the heat, almost womblike. No one else was there, so I sat and looked out across the desert, finally opening my Bible to read the temptation scene again. Satan's first temptation was for Jesus to turn stones into bread to relieve his own hunger. The lesson of humility. For the second temptation, Satan whisked Jesus away to Jerusalem and the top of the Temple and told Jesus to throw himself off because surely angels would save him. Jesus wasn't interested. The third temptation was back here on the mountain. Satan pointed to the entire world stretched out below. "It can all be yours if you bow down to me." No luck. Jesus ordered Satan out of his life.

I puzzled over what I could learn in this moment and felt a little silly; once again, my seeking self had taken me to an outlandish situation— reading the Bible on a ledge on a mountain in the desert of Palestine. The lower half of my shorts was still wet from the river. *Who does this?* I said to myself, and not in a nice way. *All your friends are back home waking up to go to work so they can put their kids through college. You are ridiculous.* But, hey, Brad, this weird, holy trip does feel right, even crucial? It does, Brad. Doesn't it? Despite the self-abuse, I knew on a deep level that I was doing exactly what I needed to. I couldn't just go with the flow.

I imagined Jesus here, next to me, with Satan promising him *everything*. I don't know what I would have done. I had less than $3,000 in my bank account. I was still taking a large cocktail of meds. I didn't know how to love or be loved. I knew my relationship with Andrea wouldn't last. I believed I didn't have what it took to be in relationship: I am too much. Too emotionally needy. And, at the same time, too fearful and avoidant. I don't know what "everything" would have been for Jesus, but for me, I would have settled for understanding who I was, how I ended up here. I would have loved to understand my story and to receive a glimpse of a path forward. And in that moment, I had none of those things.

As it turned out, Satan was still very present on this mount, or that's certainly how I felt. Had I brought him with me? The Satan residing in my own mind, my brutal inner critic. I had enough of temptation.

My head hanging low, I walked back down the trail and got back into my hot car and headed to the highway.

This trip of a lifetime was bringing more confusion than clarity.

fifteen

AMOR FATI

THE IMAGE OF LIGHT MOVING THROUGH A CRACKED-OPEN DOOR stayed with me as I left the Jordan River Valley and drove across the so-called wilderness where Jesus was said to have fasted for forty days. This wilderness, so stark, treeless, and bleached by the sun, looked nothing like I imagined it when I was a child. Back then, I pictured the white oak and scrub pine forests of the Ozark Mountains of southern Missouri and Arkansas where my family went on occasional canoe trips. The image stayed with me as I arrived at the remote and dusty turnoff to the Wadi al-Nar, Valley of Fire, Road.

I could have taken the new four-lane highway built by Israel for use only by Israelis, but I've always preferred two-lane back roads because they feel closer to nature and to humans, too. But this road was a doozy. The Valley of Fire Road is a poorly maintained, two-lane affair that climbs desert hill after desert hill and drops into steep, narrow wadis, or valleys. This rugged, rocky scenery—and the knowledge that if your car broke down here, you would find few natural or human resources to survive—evoked solitude edging toward fear, or at least an acute uneasiness. If I didn't have a long-term life plan, I did have a plan for the rest of the afternoon. I wanted to get to Bethlehem, a distance of fifty-nine miles, before the tourist sites closed. I wanted to visit the Church of the Nativity, the Milk Grotto Church, and Shepherd's Field, plus a few others. Next, I planned to continue to Checkpoint 300 near the site of Rachel's Tomb, where I knew I'd face interrogation by Israeli soldiers charged with keeping suicide bombers out of Israel. They ask predictable questions: Where are you from? Why are you here? How long will you stay? Do you know anybody in Palestine? When they speak to you, the heavily armed, flak-jacket-wearing soldiers stare so deeply into your eyes that it feels like they can actually see the thoughts floating in your head. I'd read that they are indeed trained in interpreting body language, even subtle eye movements. From there, it was an easy half-hour drive through the suburbs, with their strip-mall grocery stores and blocky two-story stone houses with xeriscape gardens, to Jerusalem, where I had a reservation at a hostel near the Old City, the historic and spiritual center, home to most of the city's religious sites.

I switched off the radio. The desert turned deep red, and I fell into a trance. I envisioned Jesus walking across this moonscape, camping near streams in the oasis-like greenery of the deep wadis, hiding from robbers and, while craving physical nourishment, finally accepting the spiritual nourishment that fasting and solitude can bring. Of course, this was the place he chose after his baptism. He needed to literally bake in his new status as a fully realized spiritual leader. He needed to integrate the first thirty years of his life as a human with his new calling as a divine human and gather his thoughts to prepare his teachings. It must have been intuition, but he knew that it wasn't enough to think or believe he was powerful. He needed to feel it in his muscle and bone, in his ligaments and organs. Especially his heart.

I considered pulling over and spending forty days here. Would that straighten me out? I imagined something like those "tough love" camps for "troubled" teens in the Utah outback. Perhaps denying myself food for a month or so would clear the cobwebs out of my head and help me find the direction and passion I knew I needed to move forward with my life—to *have* a life.

The road grew bumpier, and I had to slow down. I needed to make good time to arrive in Bethlehem by four in the afternoon. Any later, and

I might not be permitted to enter the Church of the Nativity and see the traditional site of Jesus's birth. Although I had someplace to be, I also wasn't in that much of a hurry. I had a distinct feeling that I would be coming back to Palestine. I had more to see and experience here.

The road began to bend to the south and then descended sharply. My rental car handled the roller coaster–like hills and dips just fine, but on the steep climb up the other side of the Valley of Fire, it slowed. A lot. Then the air conditioner faltered, the vents started blowing snow-flakes, and the air inside became the same temperature as the air out-side, which indeed felt like fire. I was tired and sweaty. Still, with each hairpin turn, I felt like I was waking up to a new view of my life. If I held any illusions about returning to a life as an adventure writer, they dissolved between Jericho and Bethlehem. I was in no condition to resume that career, with all its physical discomforts and possible dan-gers. Besides, the internet had wrecked the business of writing; the same publications that had paid me $10,000 for a long-form article were now offering $2,000, or $1,000, or even less. The road back to my old career was closed. The gods, the Fates, or whoever nudges us when our own willpower fails had different plans for me. I needed to accept my new fate. Perhaps I needed to love it. I was on this planet to heal. Period. I would have to find a way to support myself enough to get by in life. I needed a good therapist, a psychiatrist with a broader view of his pa-tients than Dr. Winston, a community of friends, and plenty more that I knew I wasn't aware of. Maybe I needed to move away from Santa Fe. All of this was in my mind as I drove.

When I arrived in the Holy Land a week before, I was fueled by enthusiasm and the desire to get out of the house and move through this beautiful, historic, and spiritually significant land. And to write a travel article again. And, yes, I enthusiastically hiked the Jesus Trail and en-joyed it, but I now understood that I'd walked from Nazareth to the Sea of Galilee in the same state of clueless hope that things would get better on their own. I was living in particular patterns that I'd been stuck in for decades. I hoped that hiking the Jesus Trail would reveal some new path to me, but I had no real plan on how to begin the healing process. This past week, I hadn't found the necessary humility that any major reclamation project requires; I was still an arrogant adventure writer, or what was left of one, groping for fame and fortune.

THE YEARS LEADING UP TO THIS TRIP HAD BEEN DIFFICULT FOR several reasons, but looking back, the isolation stands out most strongly to me now. Trauma causes us to see danger where it's not always present—and this includes in other people. When I met somebody new, I either trusted them too easily—so that I allowed virtual strangers, particularly women, to get too close too soon. With men, I feared their aggression. I became paranoid that they had ulterior motives to hurt me or that I couldn't trust them to tell me the truth, like my dad. So I isolated myself. And when we isolate ourselves, we tend to get trapped in a prison of our thoughts, which can be off base or even wildly incorrect. And since humans are wired for connection, I also didn't experience the calming effect that friends can provide. I could no longer turn to my family. Since I was divorced and had no kids, I hadn't created a family of my own that I could lean on. Since I left the staff at *Outside* and started working on my own, I didn't have a community of colleagues. Andrea and I had a sweet connection, but we were both suffering from trauma, and that created problems, too. I was trapped in what David Foster Wallace called "our little skull-shaped kingdom."

My path was not clear to me, yet I knew I needed one. And I understood that a path can be spiritual practice, a vision for our lives, or even a hobby that makes us feel enthused and alive. At first, my work and psychiatry had been my path, and for a while that was somewhat sustaining. And although the medications' numbing properties likely kept me alive during the most challenging times, they hadn't given me any sense that I was on a sustainable path of healing. I was overly reliant on my doctor and the pharmaceutical industry, just waiting for the next best pill to hit the market that might "fix" me. The psychiatry path fed nihilism. *My life will never get better,* I had told myself, so I kept taking pills and hoped for the best.

As I forged a path on this trip, I was seeking new ways of seeing myself other than as a bipolar former adventure writer who'd dropped out of society. I was chasing spirituality for a very sound reason: I had been holding a tiny, limited view of myself as a collage of diagnoses. And living as a diagnosis—as a more or less passive patient—is no way to live. Spirituality promised a bigger view of myself. Most spiritual and religious traditions offer similar benefits: peace, connection to the divine, community, meaning. These promises are hugely attractive, especially when we are fragmented, traumatized, and lost.

The impulsive trip to Qasr el Yahud and the soak in the Jordan had knocked something loose in my psyche and showed me something that I was just now—as I climbed past wrecked, abandoned cars whose drivers had lost control on the steep road—able to access. Nobody is more on fire for spirituality than a former addict trying to right the ship of their life. I wanted to be a child of God again. I wanted to feel—in my body, not just in my mind—that I was connected to others and the whole of the universe.

A flash of memory came to me.

Sophomore year in high school, the time when my life took a sharp downward turn. During the previous year, in ninth grade, I'd been my usual straight-A self. I was the confident captain of the basketball team, student body president, and winner of the Most Likely to Succeed and Most Inspirational Student trophies. But that summer had been hard. My father's drinking intensified. My mother shared with me about his long-term affair, something I'd already figured out. I comforted her as she asked me whether I thought she should leave my father. Eventually, he moved out. And then he moved back in. And then out again. I told myself and others I was fine. I kept getting straight As. I continued smiling. But I wasn't fine. I was crashing. I stopped sleeping. I had, almost overnight, lost my teenage musculature and was now skinny, anxious, and depressed. And yet we were supposed to pretend to both friends and strangers that we were a perfect American family.

A saving grace was my new friend Dee, one of the adult leaders of a Bible study group I'd attended in junior high. Later, in high school, Dee and I drove to Colorado together for a short ski trip. I felt a brotherly bond with him. We were both sensitive and spiritually inclined. On the drive home, he told me he had applied to seminary, and I was fascinated. It sounded like something I might be interested in. To go study spiritual things in school. To have a life built around spirituality and helping people connect with spirituality. I told my family about Dee's plans at the dinner table. My brother and father laughed. They mocked his name as being unmasculine. They made fun of how meek and soft-spoken he was when he picked me up in his rusty Ford Pinto. I wanted to defend Dee and my friendship with him. I now wish I had been capable of that. But I froze. I felt my face flush with shame, and then I felt sick to my stomach. I picked up my plate and set it in the kitchen and hurried to the bathroom and vomited.

I walked away from dinner doubting my friendship with Dee and determined not to spend more time with him. I feel sad that I allowed harsh, alpha-male mockery to affect how I viewed Dee, whom I never saw again. I also never revisited the idea of seminary. Of course, I would have made a horrible, doubt-filled minister, and I'd never have lasted as a faithful fundamentalist Christian. But in that moment at the dinner table, when my feelings of joy about my new friendship turned instantly to toxic shame, I shoved aside the truly spiritual side of myself and what I wanted to be and become as a person. Was that the moment when I, an introspective, spiritual young man, abandoned myself in pursuit of more traditional masculinity and a career I thought would please my father and brother? Had I, in that moment at the table, fatefully stuffed down my deep connection with God, the universe, or inner truth? These small moments, these tiny interactions, can be wrong turns we spend decades trying to reroute.

The splinter of light coming through that cracked door was telling me that healing was my fate. And I believed spirituality—adopting a bigger view of myself and the universe—was how I would fulfill that fate, but I didn't yet know what it would look like. Following Jesus was the closest thing I'd known to being spiritual so far in my life, and I was now literally walking in his footsteps, searching for a beam of light and hope that started within me that I could call my own. Could Jesus carry the cross of my shame? I knew I had a lot of hard work ahead, but I couldn't imagine the outcome. I didn't know how long it would take to get to a place that felt healed, mostly healed, even somewhat healed. This I knew: at a minimum, it would take hours, weeks, months, years of therapy. Maybe it would be the work of my life. My mind had some painful knots to unravel, and the tightest knot of all was this: Could I be more than a psych patient? Was I anything other than my diagnosis?

Suddenly, my experience in Qasr el Yahud looked like the most important thing that had ever happened to me. The door that had been slammed shut over the dinner table was opening again, and I knew that I should move through it. "The door is round and open, don't go back to sleep" is my favorite line of Rumi's poetry, though the door looked neither round nor open then. It doesn't matter that I didn't know what was coming or how long the road would be: that day, I saw a sliver of light coming through the door. Later, I'd see the doorknob and grab it. Later still, I'd tentatively pull the door open so that I could stick my head out for a better look-see. And later still, I would pull the door open and step across the threshold to the other side, into the light, into clarity, into healing, into my heart. Jesus and pills had brought me this far. I knew the pills weren't going to take me much further, and I wasn't sure about Jesus either. But when I read the Bible growing up, Jesus's gentle, loving courage, and his blend of radicalism and heart, appealed to me. His message—the way he moved through the world—was a start.

I headed up, up, up, making whiplash-like motions with the steering wheel to navigate the hairpin turns. I saw the steel and tar-paper shacks and barns of the Bedouins and their animals. My car struggled to climb, and I pressed harder on the accelerator. It was like those old arcade games I played in the 1970s and '80s where you sit in a lifelike car seat with a stick shift and navigate a cartoon road on a video screen. In the distance was a sprawling olive grove. Half of it had recently burned to the ground during a conflict between Jewish settlers and Palestinian locals. Behind me the landscape looked like an ocean of white-gold waves formed by successive layers of rolling hills. And, of course, the massive, forty-foot-high concrete Separation Wall, circling the West Bank in a motion that reminded me of a boa constrictor and just as intimidating. I passed a woman wearing a long, black cloak, a man wearing khaki trousers and a black-and-white checkered keffiyeh. They were carrying a large, clear plastic container full of water that sloshed with each strained, exhausted step.

The road finally leveled out. I passed occasional brick houses and stores—one painted with a mural of Yasser Arafat—until Google Maps led me to downtown Bethlehem. I parked the car and climbed out. It was a chilly, late afternoon up there in the mountains. The winter sun was descending behind the buildings. The Church of the Nativity was about to close for the day. I wasn't disappointed; I knew I'd be back. I found myself walking toward the intimidating, graffiti-covered Separation Wall, which runs smack through the center of Bethlehem, casting a cold, dark shadow on the street—and practically over the entire town. I stood in the cool, gray light in front of these words, painted in big, black, block letters on the wall: "NOW THAT YOU HAVE SEEN, YOU ARE RESPONSIBLE."

Farther to the right, I recognized a mural depicting a small girl holding a balloon. She was floating skyward, as if she might fly away to freedom. Another mural of a young girl frisking a heavily armed soldier. I knew the latter two to be the work of the internationally famous artist Banksy. In the weird, low light of dusk, breathing the cake-like, exhaust-choked air, I contemplated the hatred between Jews and Arabs, two Semitic cultures that shared the stories and lineage of Abraham, that had led to the wall and the deaths of thousands of Israelis and Palestinians in decade after decade of conflict.

My thoughts turned to a much smaller conflict, one I knew I could better understand: the conflict within my family. I knew the way forward was to walk away from blaming them for my unhappiness. I'd heard spiritual teachers say countless times that resentment only hurts the person who holds it. I needed to let go of my anger at my father for the toxic shame that consumed me and which I believed was borne of his drinking and betrayals. I wanted to let go of my anger at my brother for his cruel remarks, bullying, and dismissiveness. I desired to forgive my mother for failing to protect us, just kids, from my father's destructiveness. It was too much anger to hold. As much as I needed to do this work, I also knew that it would be a process, long and likely confusing and taxing. But I could—I would—do it. I took a deep breath of the chilly air, and I walked back to Manger Square. Although this trip was definitely not going to re-Christianize me, the Bible said that the town I found myself in was the place where God sent his Son to take human form and absolve human beings of our sins. I wished it was going to be that simple for me. I knew it wasn't, but in the chilling air and with a rumble in my stomach, just the idea of a fresh start was comforting.

After dinner at an outdoor shawarma shack, I climbed back into my car and passed through the stiff security at Checkpoint 300. It was nerve-racking, but I was too tired to care. I calmly answered the soldiers' questions as they swept the undercarriage of my rental for bombs. I drove along Highway 60, turned left onto Chopin Street, and found myself fighting traffic on Sultan Suleiman Avenue and entering Jerusalem on its Arabic eastern side. The Arabic neighborhoods, filled with nondescript, blocky, water-tank-topped apartments, and tiny grocery stores and cafes marked by signs in their curvy script, were quiet. My own breath, on the other hand, was ear-splittingly loud.

I felt wonder and nostalgia. Here I was in the three-dimensional magical land that up to this point had existed only on the page and in my youthful imagination. I was also experiencing a visual and emotional flashbacks to those hard times of my youth, which had warped my mind and physical brain. I read so much about Jerusalem as a kid, and I had held a picture of it in my mind based on what I'd read, mental images that both resembled and didn't resemble what I was seeing now. The streets, made of asphalt instead of dirt, swarmed with buses and cars, and the people wore T-shirts and pants. It wasn't peaceful at all. After the highs and lows of my experiences at the Jordan and the Mount of Temptation, I was now energized by delight, surprise, and familiarity; I sat lower in my seat, trying to stay grounded so that I didn't fly out of my car window in some ecstatic, Rapture-like explosion.

Sultan Suleiman Avenue was named for Suleiman the Magnificent, the sixteenth-century leader of the Ottoman Empire, which controlled Palestine for four hundred years until the British occupied it in 1917. As I rambled down the street, the Old City came into view. The walls were lit up by floodlights, giving the blond limestone—the building blocks of ancient and modern buildings from King David's time to now—a ghostly pale glow. Covering only 224 acres, the Old City, located on the dividing line between Arabic East Jerusalem and Israeli/Jewish West Jerusalem, is the city's spiritual center. It looked like a fortress, and that's precisely what it was. The forty-foot walls have been built and rebuilt many times; those standing today were constructed by Suleiman. But my eye was quickly drawn by the gold Dome of the Rock, the famous Muslim shrine, and then to two other impressive landmarks: Al-Aqsa Mosque, with its soft gray-black dome, and on the west side, the Church of the Holy Sepulchre, as tall as the Dome of the Rock but less ostentatious, with its muted blue tiles. City of David Street took me along the Valley of Josephat, where the Old Testament says God will gather and judge all nations.

The eastside walls were to my right, and the Mount of Olives, now mostly cleared of olive trees, replaced by ancient and modern graves, was on my left. I gazed up at this hill that lived larger in my imagination than any other far-off place in the world. At one point in my teenage obsession with Jesus, I fell under the spell of Hal Lindsey, the apocalyptic fundamentalist author of *The Late Great Planet Earth*. This book, which sold millions of copies in the 1970s, proclaimed that the End Days would arrive soon, likely within the decade. First, the Rapture would occur, when those who met the criteria of being "good Christians" would disappear from the earth and be zoomed up to heaven, leaving steaming shoes and clothes and any other baggage of life on earth behind. I couldn't believe

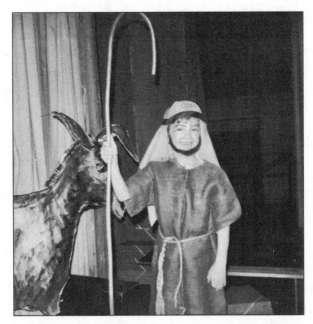

I must have been around eight years old when I played a shepherd in the Christmas pageant at St. Michael's Church in Mission, Kansas.

I was here. And I couldn't believe I had believed all that. And I loved science class back then, too.

As I became a teenager, I spent little time with my father except at night when he was drunk or Sundays when we went to church as a family. My mother seemed to be MIA, too. She always seemed to have another meeting to attend. Yet another group had elected her to be their president. I leaned more heavily on the teachings of Jesus, which I interpreted through Lindsey's inflammatory words and rigid, apocalyptic, doomsday worldview. Without much fatherly guidance, I went down a religious rabbit hole of my mind's creation. My inner critic became more and more bullying until it was like an angry God inside my head, and my thinking became obsessive and delusional. I felt toxic, and I feared I would infect others. I began to worry that I could impregnate a woman by kissing them. I feared I might give somebody AIDS, though I'd never even had sex with anybody. I doubled down on trying to purify myself. I tried to give up masturbating and scolded myself when I failed. I told myself I was sinful for making out at a party with a girl in my class whom I liked. I attempted to Christianize my behavior in the warped way that only a teenager under the spell of fundamentalism could. My goal: qualify for the Rapture.

According to Lindsey, those humans left behind on earth would experience terrifying times after the Rapture. As foretold in the book of Revelation, the Antichrist would appear. A prominent political or economic leader would plunge the planet into chaos. World War III would break out, and there would be fierce battles worldwide, including in Israel. As the earth heated up, Jesus would finally return in the sky in dramatic form over the Mount of Olives. He would fly right over where I was driving now and enter Jerusalem through the Golden Gate, one of the seven gates leading into the Old City, which was currently walled up.

I turned left on Jaffa Street, passing Hebrew University and several open-air cafes, and then began looking for my hostel at 67 HaNaviim Street. The roads were so silent, they seemed abandoned—except for a Haredim man wearing a long frock, a long beard, side curls, and a top hat, walking earnestly along. I admired and felt a bit envious of his purposeful march. He looked like he had a spiritual connection, a spiritual meaning, a spiritual life—though I couldn't articulate what that meant or might look like for me. I didn't know what I was hungry for, I just knew I was hungry. But I knew now that I had to be careful with what I did to satisfy that hunger.

I HAD A reservation at Abraham Hostel, run by a progressive Jewish businessman named Maoz Inon, one of the founders of the Jesus Trail. I found a place to park on the street, grabbed my backpack, entered, and checked in at the front desk. My room was spare: a single bed, white tile floor, and air conditioner. I was exhausted from the long drive and the heat, and I was somehow dusty and wet at the same time.

After a shower, I paused to look at myself in the mirror. I had turned forty-six three weeks earlier, just a few days before leaving for this trip. I looked younger, somehow, and inside I felt almost boyish. Or rather like I was still fifteen, full of that angsty mix of naivete and bravado. Anxious to leave childhood and find out what's supposed to come next. Despite all that I'd been through—the world travel, the kidney damage, the drugged-out years I was trying to emerge from—I looked young, albeit still a little puffy in the face from the drugs. I stood six feet tall and weighed in the 190s. There was a gut pushing out over the top of my pants. *I need to get back into shape*, I thought.

As I stared at my reflection, I thought about a mystifying encounter with Jesus I'd had in my bathroom when I was about fifteen. One night, during a long period of sleeplessness, I crawled out of bed, where my mind had been anxiously spinning stories. As I entered the bathroom, I caught my own reflection in the mirror. I had been losing weight due to an anxious stomach, and I looked bony and a little gaunt. Weak, scared, with dark circles under my eyes. At first, I saw myself in the mirror. But as I stared more closely, I became confused about who or what I was looking at. I spoke to the man-boy in the mirror. *Who are you?* I said. *Who are you?* I watched my lips speak the words. I heard them through my ears. I don't know how to explain what happened next. It was delusion bordering on psychosis. But spun differently it was also beautiful, meaningful. It might have been me, my wiser self, assuring me I was not the feeble, scared boy I believed myself to be. And who knows? Maybe some part of us really is divine, like Jesus, like the yogis of India say. But I swear on the Bible that the man-boy standing in front of the mirror in his tighty-whities answered my question with these words: *Am I Jesus? Am I Jesus? . . . I am Jesus.*

I know this story is weird and perhaps shocking. You might be thinking that this story proves that I was mentally ill, seriously mentally ill, then and now. And I have no doubt that this episode, when I retold it to my first psychiatrist, did contribute to my bipolar diagnosis. But I assure you that this merging of boy and God was quite temporary. I woke up as Brad, and I have remained Brad for the past fifty-six years. How do I see it now? Of course, it's dissociative. And trauma causes dissociation. It was also a gift from the gods or whoever grants such spiritual gifts. In a family that was confusing and difficult to be part of, I had some way of seeing myself as more than a weak, scared, depressed boy.

Of course, this man looking in the mirror in Jerusalem no longer looked boyish. I noticed my midsection, no longer as taut as it was even five years before. My mind turned to yoga, which I had quit doing when I fell into the walking drug coma. Maybe I was craving it again—the movement, the way I felt when I practiced consistently. Yoga used to bring me closer to peace than most anything else. I felt calm and in balance with myself after a yoga class, when my nervous system was able to settle, even if only for a short time. I would resume my yoga practice when I returned home. I had a few more crow's feet, and there were flecks of gray in my hair and beard, but I was still here, still searching.

I was also still taking five medications, which I tipped methodically, one by one, into my hand and washed down with a palmful of water from the sink. I did this every morning and night, no matter how tired I was or how late I was running. It was my ritual, my constant, my blood brother. I had already considerably reduced the number of pills I took regularly, and it would take a lot of work to get off the rest. I wondered if I could do it. But I was getting ready for it, I told myself.

After the chemical Holy Eucharist, I collapsed into bed.

I would learn over the following years to see my overmedication as an addiction issue. I didn't know how to cope with my feelings of anger and emptiness. Maybe it was my religious orientation, but beyond marijuana and a few experiences with psychedelics, I had stayed away from street drugs. If I hadn't been so paranoid and worried about my status and reputation as a writer, I imagine I would have loved cocaine. Instead, I got my drugs from a doctor. My pusher did look a little bit like Jesus, but he wore a white coat and went to medical school. I thought he would save me.

Still too jagged from the day's adventures in Palestine to sleep, I took out the book I'd brought with me, *The Gnostic Gospels*, by Elaine Pagels.

I was fascinated to learn about these other accounts of Jesus that had been discovered across the Middle East: the gospels of Thomas, Mary Magdalene, and Judas. Pagels and others argued that the early church, which quickly became a political organization when Rome embraced it, was forced to select which Scriptures to include in the New Testament, the texts that would become canonical, acceptable, the texts to offer wisdom and guidance. It was disappointing, yet unsurprising, that the chosen texts were those that served the purposes of the ruling class; the texts that were excluded held opinions and stories that endangered the ruling class, and they were banned. These disgraced Gnostic Gospels might have been closer to how an iconoclastic Jesus taught. *Gnosis* means "knowledge or inner knowing," and the Gnostic Gospels suggested that Jesus, who lived inside each of us, could be accessed by plumbing the depths of our psyche, our soul, our spirit, which held knowledge that transcended our physical form. Contemplative activities like meditation and prayer could take you inward to Jesus. One line from the gospel of Thomas spoke to me as I read it on my hostel bed: "If you bring forth what is within you, what you bring forth will save you. If you do not bring forth what is within you, what you do not bring forth will destroy you."

Whatever was remaining inside of me *was* killing me, slowly. Yes, the pills, the resentment, the anger. But also me! The good version of Brad that I had lost touch with decades ago. This Brad was screaming at me, "Let me out!" But how to get it out? Or how to get *me* out?

I set down the book, realizing that I was at the tip of an iceberg, and I was the iceberg. I wasn't in Israel to write a story about the Jesus Trail and go home. I was on a pilgrimage—in the midst of a religious act, on a journey to visit holy places, pay homage, and fortify my faith, whatever that might look like. *I will write the* Times *article in a few weeks*, I said to myself. *For now, I am a pilgrim. A pilgrim with no particular religion, god, or guru.*

I figured it was early afternoon in Santa Fe, and I decided to text Andrea. I didn't want her to worry, and I also didn't feel like texting anything about my intense experiences over the past few days. Still, I wrote:

Hi, Sweetie, I'm in Jerusalem now. I had an interesting day. I'll tell you more later. I just checked into my hostel. I'll call you tomorrow. Love, Brad.

The sun hadn't set yet, but the meds were working their magic, and I fell quickly asleep.

Sleep didn't last long.

My own screams woke me from a dream. An underwater dream. A nightmare. I was consumed by the terror and the weird blend of realness and otherworldliness with which nightmares take over our sleeping minds.

I am swimming at the bottom of a deep body of water, maybe the ocean. I am wearing glasses, but everything is foggy. I can feel the bottom, the sand, small rocks, and shells, but no matter how close I get, I can't see. I swim along like I'm floating in outer space, not knowing where I'm headed, and then I realize I am underwater, and I can't breathe. I wake up enough to realize that I am dreaming, but I am still sleeping, too. I realize that I've stopped breathing in real life. I try to inhale but my body won't take a breath. What little air remains in my lungs, I force out and try to emit a shout. But since I'm still asleep, my voice is stuck in my throat. I push harder with the air in my lungs. I begin to hear through my ears a warped, ungodly moan, and my eyes open to realize I made the moan. I open my lungs and air rushes in, and I lie there, breathing deeply and rapidly. Adrenaline and fear fill my torso and limbs. As the breathing slows, I relax.

It was dark out. I looked at my phone. 4:45. *Shit. Not again.* For months I'd been waking at this time, not usually from a nightmare, but I couldn't sleep beyond five. I lay there for a few minutes until I accepted that I wasn't going back to sleep. I rose and went downstairs to make a cup of instant coffee. I might as well go down to the Old City and poke around in the streets and buildings where Jesus spent his final week alive.

I drank my coffee. I understood that my life had entered a new phase. *Pilgrim* sounded nice if a tad hopeful given that I had spent my savings on this trip and would need to go home to make some money. *Patient.* I hoped not. I stopped trying to come up with a label and walked out the door onto HaNaviim Street—the Street of the Prophets.

I meandered around the north side of the Old City, past the bus station and an outdoor bazaar, to Damascus Gate, the beginning of the road to Damascus, famous as the site of the conversion of Paul the Apostle. The architecture was medieval—gargoyles and all. Of the seven gates into the Old City, the Damascus Gate is the oldest, and the only entrance that has kept its Arabic name. The gate itself is a conglomeration of architectural styles, a mashup of ancient Roman columns, Middle Eastern pyramids, and medieval Ottoman semidomes. It also looks most like a traditional entrance to a fortified castle. The trimmings around the opening are for defensive purposes, not for decoration or show. The turret is interrupted by crenellations, strategically placed openings where soldiers could shoot arrows or hurl projectiles. There are machicolations, protected openings where soldiers could dump boiling oil or lime on attackers, and more screaming gargoyles. It was quiet at this time of morning, but, later in the day, I would experience this place as a bustling, noisy, vibrant marketplace. Tiny speakers mounted on long sticks emitted tinny, celebratory Arab music, which blended in with the shouts of vendors selling everything from children's underwear to falafel.

Descending the stairs, I walked through the void-like opening. There wasn't a soul around.

I walked across this threshold alone, which seemed right. Nothing changed, but everything changed. Label or no label, I was conscious of my life's purpose—at least for now. Not a pilgrim, not a seeker, but a man who was finding the humility and strength to heal. I was stepping into a new world, and that new world was inside me.

The door is round and open, don't go back to sleep.

sixteen

JERUSALEM

I KNOW I AM NOT ALONE IN HAVING BEEN CALLED AN *OLD SOUL* AT a young age—many of us seem and feel wise beyond our years. Growing up in Kansas in the 1970s, I certainly behaved like a typical kid in many ways, not like a seasoned monk in a monastery. But in my early teens, I noticed that I seemed to be more sensitive than other boys. I liked sports, and I was good at them, and I liked other typical boy stuff, too, but after the ball playing was over, I wanted to talk about emotions and about psychological and spiritual matters.

By age thirteen, I noticed new ways my sensitivity was showing up. On sunny days, I felt bright and hopeful. On cloudy days, I felt contemplative and moody. When I sat in my room reading books and listening to music that was emotionally intense, I felt like I was merging with the words and sound, and maybe the artist, too. When I first read Jack Kerouac's *On the Road*, I felt euphoric, like the fast-driving, fast-talking, speed-taking Dean Moriarty character took over my body. I practiced speaking like him in beatific, stream-of-consciousness style. The first time I listened to Jimi Hendrix's "All Along the Watchtower," I became the swirling guitar solo. The song evoked every emotion inside me. The feeling circled in my torso and up and down my limbs, like a beautiful firestorm. Tears welled in my eyes. And, of course, when I read about Jesus, I experienced similar feelings. I wanted to be him, I formed his words in my mouth over and over, and I practiced holding my body erect, with shoulders back, while also keeping my heart soft, in a way I thought he might have.

I always saw this proclivity, this desire to merge as a blessing, a gift. But it could feel too intense sometimes, too. And then, seven years after my Holy Land pilgrimage, after I was diagnosed with childhood trauma, PTSD, and complex PTSD, I learned about the effects that adverse childhood experiences can have on our adult personalities. And it turns out, my special skill was one of those effects.

Studies show that children who experience traumatic events—like my near drowning but also the ongoing traumas of growing up in a dysfunctional, toxic family—are permanently changed. Unsurprisingly, these children suffer more depression, but trauma also changes their personalities in a specific way: they tend to score high in what psychologists call *openness*. Openness is a quality of being more vulnerable, impressionable, and receptive to ideas, experiences, creativity, novelty, and—get this—thrill seeking. Although all of this may sound like a good thing, and it can be, openness has a shadow side. We can become too trusting. We can have weak boundaries and underdeveloped discernment about danger. We can be oblivious to manipulative, even dangerous, people. And, of course, this often leads us to being further traumatized when our curiosity leads us into situations beyond our control. A sadly classic example is when those who suffer from the trauma of sexual abuse find themselves seeking risky situations involving sex. For me? During my adventure-writing years, I was too trusting of strangers. I was unafraid to engage with them, and I shared too much. When I was on the road, like Dean Moriarty, I felt wide open and ready for anything. Ready to merge with the world. Desperate to escape into the next stranger's arms. This confusion about where I ended and others began was usually short lived, but oh God did it feel marvelous. I craved escape like a drug.

Today, when I look back at my time in the Holy Land, I now see the whole trip was an attempt to re-create my youthful merging with Jesus. As I entered the Old City on that frosty February morning, I was seeking the Jesus of my youth. I wasn't merely trying to understand who he was in real life, or even who he was in the Gospels; I was trying to onboard him into my psyche, into my very soul. I breathed in the cold, dark air, trying to settle my nervous system so that I could feel. Feel what? Feel everything. And nothing. Everything of Jesus and nothing of my own pain. And like a spiritualist who places her hands on a table and calls in the spirit of a deceased loved one, I summoned Jesus. I muttered no words of prayer. I wasn't meditating on his image or his name; I was emptying my own self out, hoping that I'd never come back.

The sound of my shoes against the paving stones echoed down the empty street as I disappeared into the dimly lit Muslim Quarter. Utterly deserted at this hour, my breath was the only other sound. In less than an hour, these narrow, covered streets would be lined with high-energy vendors selling hibiscus, oregano, and cardamom from old baskets; freshly butchered lamb and pork, golden loaves of bread just out of the oven; and red, yellow, and orange sweets piled up in mounds. But now, in the predawn quiet, I felt like I had walked into a dream, the thick, all-too-vivid type that seems more real than waking life. In such dreams, you know the images are meant to teach you something, but you don't know how to make sense of them. Pink neon store signs clashed with the cold, gray stone. I didn't need a map. I'd been studying one for weeks, and I memorized the locations of the crucial Jesus sites.

My intent was to disappear, to merge with both history and myth, and see what happened. I did need a strong cup of coffee, so I kept my eye out for a cafe that might be ready to open. I passed a butcher shop window where a whole pig carcass hung from a rusty hook through its snout. Next, I spotted a baker rolling out pastry dough on a wood counter. An older Palestinian woman wearing a traditional brightly colored blue, white, green, and yellow dress sat on the street, pulling herbs from bags to display for sale on her lap.

I turned left at the Via Dolorosa, the Way of Pain, the route Jesus walked with the cross on his way to Golgotha. As the street sloped steeply, I felt like the survivor of a capsized ship, wandering the upside-down hallways trying to figure out which way was up. Soon I was no longer alone. Vendors were arriving to set up shop. I approached a Palestinian man wearing a black stocking cap warming his hands over a copper pot.

"Coffee?" I asked.

"Yes, sir. Just two or three more minutes."

His name was Ibrahim, and we chatted while he poured sugar and cardamom into the open pot. The concoction bubbled as he stirred. He grabbed a long handle and poured the hot, sweet mixture into a tiny blue porcelain coffee cup. I traded the cup for a ten-shekel coin and stepped to the side to take the first sip, which was delicious and strong, the perfect combination of bitter and sweet. He asked me where I was from, and I told him.

"Christian?"

"Yes." I didn't want to explain to another person that I was on the fence—agnostic or something like it, although I felt a resistance to labels in general. In this part of the world, everybody belongs to some religion. As my coffee cooled, I drank bigger sips, and when I reached the mud-like grounds at the bottom, I smiled and thanked him and returned the cup to a silver tray.

"Goodbye, Ibrahim. I hope business is good today."

"Inshallah," he said. *God willing.*

The streets of the Old City were coming alive with pilgrims: Christians, Muslims, Jews. European tour groups, couples, and a few solo pilgrims. The Haredim men walked fastest. They were on their way to pray at the Western Wall, the holiest spot in the world for Jews. I ran my hand along the limestone walls as I walked on, just to make sure this experience wasn't a dream. I noticed I wasn't the only person doing this. The cold stone reminded me of the cold stone walls of St. Michael and All Angels Episcopal Church, where, on more than a few cold winter mornings, I served as an acolyte at the early 7 a.m. service.

At the Via Dolorosa again, I turned right and headed east. I passed through an arch, St. Stephen's Gate, also known as Lion's Gate, and found myself outside the city walls. I knew this place well. Here the apostle Stephen, found guilty of blasphemy, was stoned to death. The sun felt warm on my skin. After only a few more steps, I reached the Tomb of the Virgin, the traditional site of Mary's tomb, and descended the steep stairs into the nave, which reminded me of a cave, womb-like. Mary's death isn't mentioned in the Bible, but Eastern Christians revere this place as the location where the mother of Jesus was buried and, later, ascended to heaven, where Jesus is believed to have met her. I thought about my own strong beliefs in Jesus when I was a teenager, and my hope—no, my anxiety—around whether I had lived a pure enough life for Jesus to meet me in heaven should I die young. Some days I was convinced I'd qualify. On other days, I felt too much shame around my changing body and even my compulsive people pleasing. When I was compliant, I felt conflicted inside. It felt right and good to keep adults happy. My parents couldn't stand hearing if I slipped up and a teacher or another parent was unhappy with me. I felt so ashamed of myself, even if the adult was actually in the wrong. "What did you do to deserve it, Brad?" my mom would say. But at the same time, being obsequious to adults felt shitty inside. Like I was betraying myself. And I figured that God didn't like bullshit people pleasing either. So, I often felt trapped. Same with my dad's drinking: If I said something, he got angry, and my mother did too. I was accused of being disrespectful. But if I said nothing? It felt worse. I knew I was stuffing down my truth, and I went to bed fuming. It was a classic double bind. No matter what I did, I felt bad.

I emerged from the Tomb of the Virgin, blinking in the strong sunlight before crossing Jericho Road. Walking through an open gate led me into a fenced garden of massive, gnarled olive trees: the Garden of Gethsemane. It was mind-boggling to be in the very garden where Jesus faced the reality of his imminent death. I placed my hand on the bark of the biggest, thickest olive tree and held it there. The tree's massive, gnarled trunk reminded me of how grounded Jesus seemed throughout his difficult life. Long before I knew what the word "scapegoat" meant, I had seen Jesus as the scapegoat of the society in which he lived. He had no earthly father. Joseph was merely a stand-in. His real Father was just a hypothetical one who lived in a far-off imaginary place called heaven.

Was father hunger the reason Jesus became a truth teller? And, man, he was good at it. So much better than I was. He had no fear when speaking truth to power. He reminded both the Jewish elite and the Romans of their hypocrisy, their greed, and the emptiness of commerce-based spirituality. He stood his ground. He accepted the outcome of his rebellion. And yet he had doubts. I loved reading about his doubt. The Gospel of Mark, the original Gospel, and one that does not include the resurrection story, describes Jesus's last night in Garden of Gethsemane, where he prayed to God, his Father. He asked his disciples to stand guard while he meditated. In an emotional appeal in which his sweat turned to blood, he asked, "Father, if you are willing, please take this cup of suffering away from me. Yet I want your will to be done, not mine." Fuck, I thought. That doubt-filled moment when he cried a tear and asked God to stop the insanity and save him happened right here where I was now standing. I felt the edge of another emotional flashback. I was now wrapping my arms around the trunk and leaning my torso against the rough bark, pressing my own heart into the old, gnarly olive trunk. His own fucking Father hung him out to dry. I left Gethsemane, shaking my head in awe of his openhearted courage. If only I could be as openhearted and courageous. Then I could pull my life together. Maybe I could find a new career, a new path in which I could use the gifts of my own heart instead of my arrogance.

I left Gethsemane wrapped up in my memories of my late-night Bible-reading jags from childhood. Only three other places from the New Testament lived as large as Gethsemane in my mind: Golgotha, the rock on which Jesus was crucified; the Temple Mount, where Jesus raged at the money changers; and the Mount of Olives. And now, as the morning sun grew hotter, I was right at the foot of the iconic place, a broad mountain east of the Old City where the book of Acts states Jesus ascended to heaven. I entered through the cemetery's gate and walked up the steep path toward the summit. I hadn't done much uphill hiking in a while, and the path was steep. I was alone except for a man digging a new grave with a yellow backhoe. I gazed up at the wide open sky.

There were only a few small puffy clouds. As I got closer to the top, I felt a wave of sadness, and the past flooded my mind and body until I could no longer distinguish the two. I was consumed by a PTSD flashback. I pictured my fourteen-year-old self, a straight-A people pleaser by day, left alone to watch over his drunk father into the evening, who went to bed praying desperately for the Rapture to come. The sadness—feeling now what that teenager was too scared to acknowledge, let alone feel, the truth of my painful childhood—grew until it filled my chest. Grief about the months and years compromised by depression, smiling, pretending that I felt fine, but betraying myself and the truth. The years spent over-medicated on the couch staring at the ceiling, feeling numb to the world, unable to write or even relate to my own wife. This grief felt pointed and specific but also ancient and bottomless and maybe not really about me, as the sorrow I felt came from humanity's ocean of heartbreak.

Finally, I reached the top of the Mount of Olives, or as high as the cemetery fence allowed. I turned and looked down at the Old City's maze of ancient streets and houses, the auric Dome of the Rock and the more subtle but equally impressive shrines and monuments. I saw the ant-like pilgrims from all corners of the world moving through the streets, touching the stone walls, praying at the Western Wall. I thought about who they were and why they were here. What brought them to God's door? What flavor of suffering were they experiencing? What abuses from family, strangers, or government officials had they endured? What accidental injuries to body and mind and spirit—car wrecks, floods, wildfires, and other forces beyond their control—had they faced? What stories of the ancient scriptures that grew from this harsh desert land spoke to them and offered them a hint of freedom? How had these cobblestone streets convinced them they'd find relief, refuge, even liberation by dropping their daily duties and cares and coming here to wander and pray? Were their heads filled with similar self-abusive thoughts? Were their bodies weighed down with shame?

And then I looked up at the sky again. Right there! Right above me, where that puffy cow-shaped cloud was passing over. That patch of sky is exactly where the firebrand preachers I listened to on late-night radio told me that Jesus would appear at the Second Coming. He would appear surrounded by bright light, his robes glowing like a million-watt lightbulb, his arms spread wide to embrace all of humanity. And then this hovering human-God would float across the deep, grassy valley below and enter the holy Temple Mount through the Golden Gate. Right. Fucking. There. I felt a ball of poisonous rage form in the pit of my belly and then explode into my chest. I became that scared, lonely kid again. My heart pounded against my sternum. I raised my fist to the sky. *Where the hell were you, Savior? I did my part. I prayed and read the Bible every night, sometimes till dawn. But you stood me up! You stiffed me! You didn't fucking come and take me away!*

Damn! It was too much. I breathed in deep. This pilgrimage was overwhelming me. My desire to merge with God had outstripped my ability to manage my own frayed nervous system. I felt the need to stop the feelings, the sadness, the weird elation, too. Now! I reached my arms to the sky. I formed a fist, and I shook it at nothing and everything like I did when I was sixteen and my mother told me that Dad was moving back in for a few weeks at Christmas so that Grandma and Uncle Wallace and Aunt Caryl wouldn't have to know that he had left us. And suddenly I was no longer forty-six. My body heaved, and I felt like my mind had been hijacked. By what? The past. I was no longer in the present. I was no longer me; I was the past. I was sixteen and skinny and flooded with the same anger that kept me up at night until I figured out how to stuff it down my own neck like rotten food. I stuffed it down my gullet past my stomach into the depths of my pelvis, and then I didn't stop. I stuffed all the way through my thighs, or I tried to. I wanted it outside my own body. But I know I failed. Instead of exorcising my anger, it seeped into every cell of my body. And just when I thought I actually had purged myself of it, it became deep depression and toxic self-hatred. It never left me alone. When I found a moment of success, a day of feeling good about myself, it pushed those positive feelings aside the way a beastly bouncer at a nightclub deals with out-of-control patrons. And it got in my face and scolded and berated and abused me until I fell on the couch in submission and said, *Yessir, you are right. I'm shit. You are always right, sir. Thank you for setting me straight. I'll go back to being a zero again.*

Stop! I cried. *Stop! Get out of my life, you motherfucker!*

I didn't understand what a flashback was at the time. When the past became the present and I had all the emotional maturity of a sixteen year old, I first became confused. And then I wanted to scream. I hated myself. *This is exactly why your family can't stand you, Brad. You're a fucking sixteen-year-old in a man's body!*

I pulled my arms back in, and, crying now, I walked back down the path, past the grave digger, past the thousands of ancient white markers. I crossed the busy street and reentered the Old City through Lion's Gate. Shoulders stooped, head tucked into my chest, I could barely look a stranger in the eye. At the first cafe I saw, I ordered bread and hummus and orange juice. I needed sustenance. I doubt food was really what I craved. But it was a start. I took out my journal to write but instead stared into space. I forgot about time. I dissociated out until the waitress grabbed my empty plate and glass and asked me whether I needed anything else. "Yeah," I said. "But I don't think you can help me. Thank you, though." I paid my bill and went back to walking the streets of the Old City. My fingers interlaced behind my back, my gaze directed at my feet, I walked and breathed. I walked and breathed. The flashback was over, and I wanted to be anywhere but inside myself. There was nothing I could do but continue walking . . . continue walking and trying to do the impossible: merge with the Jesus of my youth. As if that would solve any of my problems.

I explored the Old City all day. I stood at the Western Wall and tried to pray. I sat in a back-row pew at a small church and listened to Gregorian chanting. I dipped my hand in the Pools of Siloam, where Jewish pilgrims purify themselves before ascending to the Temple to pray. By late afternoon, I was prepared to visit the Church of the Holy Sepulchre. I knew it would be emotional, but I was already feeling a hint of overwhelm. And I supposed that was how one should feel entering the place where the divine man suffered and took his last breath.

This ghoulishly appointed cathedral with low light and shadows in every corner marks the location of two critical episodes: Jesus's crucifixion on Golgotha, the Place of the Skull, and the tomb where his body was laid to rest and from which he is said to have risen after three days. I thought about my skinny fourteen-year-old self, clad only in tighty-whities, staring into my bathroom mirror. I thought of the onset of depression around that time. The days, weeks, months, years I spent collapsed on the couch, my mind and body numb.

Inside the church, two chapels, one for Catholics and the other for Orthodox Christians, marked Calvary, the site of the crucifixion. In the Orthodox chapel I got in line behind about fifty other pilgrims and waited. When it was my turn, I stretched my hand through a carved hole in the altar and set my palm on the stone—ground zero of Jesus's death. It felt weirdly warm and sweaty. Of course it did, from the hands of the thousands of pilgrims who'd come before me. Touching that sacred stone didn't make me feel much inside, but I was glad I did it.

Descending into the central nave, I found myself in the small, sparsely decorated Adam's Chapel, named because early Christians believed Adam, the first human, according to the book of Genesis, was buried there. The chapel walls are heavy, made of ancient stone, and a Greek Orthodox altar stands in a niche at one end of the room. Behind the altar, a section of the cracked rock of Calvary is visible through a glass panel. According to tradition, an earthquake shook Jerusalem the moment Jesus died. It cracked the rock of Golgotha and ripped the veil inside the Temple. The world fell into darkness. When Jesus's blood dripped from the cross into the crack, it soaked deep into the earth, into Adam's skull. At this exact moment, all humans were redeemed.

I stood looking at the crack, puzzled by the imagery. *I wish I felt redeemed.* I wracked my brain for the hidden meaning and then asked myself why I thought there was any hidden meaning. I shamed myself.

Why the fuck are you always looking for meaning? You're torturing your-self, Brad! But I kept staring. I knew it had a message for me. I just knew. *Maybe it will come to me later.*

After a shower at my hostel, I sat at the bar in the dining area. Noa, the bartender, was a friendly Israeli woman in her twenties studying to be a psychologist. I told her about my day, and we discussed the Palestinian situation, which had motivated her to become a therapist. She explained to me that in her opinion, the younger generation of Israelis is more empathetic toward the Palestinian struggle. I met several hostel guests, a mixture of religious pilgrims of various ages and young, nonreligious travelers with around-the-world plane tickets who were spending a few days in the Holy Land. By ten o'clock, I collapsed into my bed, and by five the next morning I was back in the dining area, drinking instant coffee and eating toast before heading back to the Old City for more of my new life as a pilgrim, more attempts to merge with Jesus in some crazed, desperate hope that I would see something or feel something or get a hit of wisdom that I needed to move forward with my life.

I spent two more weeks exploring Jerusalem. By day, I wandered the Old City, visiting and revisiting biblical sites, still holding on to a magical notion that if I spent enough time soul-searching in these holy streets, I could force the issue and become a healed man. I walked to Bethany, the site of the Last Supper and the hometown of Mary, Martha, and Lazarus, whom Jesus reputedly raised from the dead. I stood inside Lazarus's tomb, or a replica of it. Here in Jerusalem, history and myth blended easily. I window-shopped for souvenirs. I was taken by a box full of crowns of thorns, but I didn't see how I would get it home on the plane.

I walked up to the Temple Mount, known to Muslims as the Haram esh-Sharif. According to both Jews and Muslims, God's presence can be felt here more than anywhere else in the Holy Land. The site of the Jewish Temple during most of the first millennium BCE, this raised plaza has been home to the Dome of the Rock and Al-Aqsa Mosque since around 700 CE. Muslims believe that the Foundation Stone, over which the shrine was built, was where God created the world as well as the first human, Adam. It is also believed to be the site where Abraham attempted to sacrifice his son, and where Muhammad's Night Journey to heaven began.

I imagined Jesus climbing the steps and topping out here amid the crowd of fellow Jews gathered to purchase animals for the priests to sacrifice as burnt offerings in the Temple. The rising smoke signaled that the sacrifice was transferred from the human realm to the holy realm. Pulsing with righteous anger, Jesus raged at the corrupt men who sold the animals. He pushed over their tables and opened the cages, releasing birds, lambs, and goats to wander freely across the plaza. "My house shall be called a house of prayer for all the nations," he said, quoting the Scriptures. "But you have made it a den of robbers." In doing so, he sealed his own fate, because after this bold act, the high priests sought to kill him. And within the week, Jesus would be captured, tried, and nailed to the cross.

As I walked, I felt another flashback coming on. And so I focused on my feet striking the paving stones and breathing, too. *Breathe, Brad. Breathe.* But the thoughts and feelings kept rising from my pelvis, and then they consumed my rib cage and pushed into my neck, up to my jaw, behind my eyes . . . and then I was gone again. I was no longer a tourist atop the Temple Mount. I was back in Kansas in the breakfast nook. My father entered the room wearing a pinstripe suit and smelling of Brut cologne. While I shoveled cereal into my mouth, he would sit at the head of the table and open the *Kansas City Star.* I spoke politely to him, of course I did. But secretly, I thought he might say something about the previous night. I thought he might apologize for passing out again and relying on my teenage body to support him on the long walk back to his bedroom, if only he could remember the night before. It would take me years, decades, to conclude that he never apologized because, in my experience, he doesn't apologize. Period. He doesn't feel shame enough to say he could have done better. And he certainly didn't apologize when somebody like me asks, no matter how gently. After so many mornings like that, the teenager could no longer sit there without wanting to walk over to him and wind up and punch him in the face and pour his breakfast over his perfectly parted hair.

The man I was on this day managed to push those old, angry thoughts back down into my gut before they highjacked my entire being. As they faded, I felt relieved. I surveyed the broad plaza, still walking with my fingers interlaced behind my back like a monk, still bowing my head, as if that posture would somehow allow me to feel holy. I tried to feel the divine up there in the one of the holiest places on earth. *Nope, I don't feel it. Not at all. Maybe some other time, I'll come back and try again.*

I LEFT THE TEMPLE MOUNT AND TOOK A SEAT IN A CAFE. OUTSIDE, Jewish boys practiced for their bar mitzvahs. A man with a long beard blew a shofar. I wrote in my journal.

Today the journals form a stack a foot high on my bookshelf. The individual passages are intense, sad, and difficult. To read them at face value is to experience a man trying to solve personal and existential problems, a man struggling to find the story of his life in order to change it.

I write about my childhood obsession with Jesus and why I think he's inspired me to travel here now. I describe the little mystical experiences. I try to make sense of what happened to my life: career, marriage, medication. At times, I write with confidence, as if I've realized something important that I'm ready to put into action. In other passages, the writing feels rudderless. Overall, it lacks a coherence you would expect from a man who spent six years working as a professional editor at an influential national magazine and a decade working as a travel and politics writer. I was so lost, and trying so hard, but still groping in the dark. I was obsessed with trying to solve the problem of my life, searching for meaning and a story about myself that I could lean on.

Today, I'm amazed that I believed any of this wandering could do anything to help me. And, you know what? Looking back, it did. All of it. Every tortured minute of it. For one thing, I was moving. I was not on the couch. Second, I was seeking wholeness and health. Call me crazy or silly or juvenile or naive, but I had faith that what I was doing there in the Holy Land would take me back home to myself. And now, a decade later, I know this: there is one thing that you must have in spades if you want to heal, faith. I'm not sure where faith comes from. Do we develop faith or is it a gift? I believe that I have always had a kernel of faith like a tiny inner sun. By whom? Fuck if I know. But it wasn't me. It wasn't mine. Instead of choosing to grow my faith in my twenties and thirties, I succumbed to chasing vivid experiences and fame until my tiny inner sun became obscured by doubt, cynicism, traumas, and the poor life choices that grew out of these things. But during these Holy Wanderings I made contact with faith again. Or maybe I needed those numbed-out years when I hit rock bottom to contact my faith again. Yes, that's it. Because faith was the entire reason I came to the Holy Land. Without it, I would never have left the couch. I would likely have used the sawed-off shotgun under the blanket in my office closet.

After five weeks of wandering around Israel and Palestine, I flew home. I embraced Andrea. But, I admit, I wasn't very present to her. I had too much on my mind. I wrote my Jesus Trail article and submitted it to the *New York Times*. I began working on a document that I hoped would eventually form a plan of action to recover my life. In late June, when the story was published, I felt a deep ambivalence. It was a fine piece of travel writing, and my editor had loved it. But as I reread it in the newspaper's print version, it seemed like a throwaway. I was struck by the same unsatisfied feeling that had haunted me during my last years as a travel writer. The story accomplished the task of taking readers on a journey to a place, and I shared the little epiphanies that this former Christian had as I hiked across the Holy Land, but somehow the writing didn't represent the experience I had. It didn't capture the deep feelings of the seeker I knew I had become. I was not an adventure writer; I was something far different. I was healing.

As spring turned to summer, I felt myself pulling away from Andrea. My nervous system was sending me mixed signals again: Was this love or danger? We met and began dating just six months after Di and I separated, and we moved in together before my divorce was finalized. Now I wasn't sure what I wanted from this relationship. Was our connection "real," or was I in a classic rebound situation? I told her I thought I should get my own apartment while I tried to make sense of all that had happened in my life over the past few months.

Andrea was understandably confused and deeply hurt. I moved into my new place feeling confused, guilty, and sad. I was in the forest, with no path in sight, even after all that work.

I couldn't stop thinking about Palestine. I called Tamer, a Palestinian tour guide and translator I met there. He had offered to host me at his family's house in the tiny village of Sawahere, just on the Palestinian side of the Separation Wall, about three miles from the Damascus Gate. As kids, his sisters used to walk to school in the Old City. I wrote up a story pitch for the *New York Times* Travel desk about being a tourist in Palestine. Forty hours later I was back in Tel Aviv.

I met a driver Tamer arranged for me. I climbed into his black Audi, and we rode westward through the flat, green coastal plane on winding roads. When the Separation Wall came into view, we skipped Qalandia for a less intense checkpoint and passed into the West Bank, past endless olive groves and gentle rolling hills.

An hour and a half later, we arrived at a walled compound. The door slid open, and we entered and parked. Tamer, a serious, bearded man in his late thirties, welcomed me into the house and showed me what would be my room for the coming days.

That afternoon, we rented a car and began two weeks of exploring. Each morning, Tamer called friends and contacts in various parts of the West Bank. He explained to me that it was always necessary to check for outbreaks of violence between Jewish settlers and locals while traveling in Palestine. We went to the Jordan River. (I didn't go in this time.) We traveled north to Nablus, south to Hebron, west to Bethlehem. Many evenings we smoked hookah and drank lemonade in the cafes of Ramallah, a forty-minute drive. Other evenings, we sat on the roof drinking arak and eating sweets in the glow of Jerusalem. We had coffee and cookies with his parents and sisters. We went to a dinner party at the home of his aunt and uncles in Dheisheh, a refugee camp south of Bethlehem, where he introduced me to a tall, thin man with a severe limp, having been shot by the Israeli army in the last intifada, in 2005.

And he took me to see the home of the youngest female suicide bomber. We walked down an alley, out onto a narrow street, and came to a small apartment made of concrete. It looked like other houses in Dheisheh except for the flowers placed at the entrance and the words painted on the wall:

Ayat al-Akhras February 20, 1985–March 29, 2002

At age eighteen, Ayat traveled by car from Dheisheh to a super-market in a trendy West Jerusalem neighborhood. There she detonated explosives she'd belted to her body, killing herself, a seventeen-year-old Israeli girl named Rachel Levy, and a fifty-five-year-old security guard named Haim Smadar, who attempted to stop her from entering the supermarket.

I breathed in deeply and exhaled with a sigh. As odious as her act of violence was, and as hard as it was to imagine, I felt that this small shrine deserved attention. Respect isn't the word. Perhaps acknowledgment of the brokenness of this land, of humankind. A holy brokenness. As I walked away from the shrine, a Palestinian boy no older than five years of age walked toward me carrying a soda bottle in his hand. He smiled at me, and then he reached back and hurled the bottle toward me. It hit the ground a couple of feet in front of me and shattered into a hundred glass shards. I turned and walked toward my car, and then Tamer and I drove back through the Valley of Fire toward his village and his home.

It took a day or two for me to lose the cloud of sadness after touring Dheisheh. Eventually, I said goodbye to Tamer and his family, and I returned to Jerusalem and my old digs at the Abraham Hostel. There, during my usual happy hour at the bar, I met two tourists from London and agreed to take them on a three-day tour of Palestine. They rented a car, and together we covered much of the territory I'd visited with Tamer. I became close with a professor from the UK named Angela, and we slept together in hotels and danced in discos in Ramallah. I told her the stories that Tamer had told me about the places we visited. She was edgy and smart. She wasn't interested as much in spiritual matters, so I turned off my seeking for a few days, and we talked about politics and philosophy. Before she left to go back to England, we went to the hostel's rooftop and sat.

"I wish we had more time to travel together," I said.

But in her mind, she was already at the airport. "Yeah, me too," she said flatly. "I wish the best for you."

We embraced, and then I returned to my room. I knew our connection had been shallow and convenient. Who doesn't want an intense weekend affair in an exotic place to take himself out of the real circumstances of life? She and I had played the same game. I enjoyed some sweet human connection, exciting sex with a relative stranger, and some laughs. And maybe that's what I needed.

I spent my last couple of days preparing for my interview with the Messiah Doctor, whom I'd missed on my first visit to Jerusalem. Lichtenberg, according to a feature I'd read in *Wired*, was the world's foremost expert on Jerusalem syndrome. The condition, which lasts from a few days to weeks and sometimes longer, afflicts Jews, Muslims, and Christians, many of them religious fundamentalists.

Jerusalem syndrome fascinated me, as I had experienced what I can only describe as a blending with Jesus when I was a kid—an experience I believed had led to my initial diagnosis of bipolar disorder. Since then, therapists have rejected the notion that those experiences indicate mental illness. In my forties, one therapist told me that 90 percent of people have some kind of mystical experience during their lifetimes. These experiences were normal, ordinary, part of the human desire to see beyond the circumstances of this life to something greater. When I told Lichtenberg in an email back in January that I was considering a book about mystical experiences such as Jerusalem syndrome, he invited me to visit him at his office at Jerusalem's Herzog Hospital.

When I arrived, I was shown to an elevator, which I took ten stories down to a clean, white hallway with a polished white tile floor and white walls. My shoes squeaked on the tile, and I heard the deep murmur of men's voices behind doors. Were they messiahs in therapy sessions?

I found Lichtenberg in his office with his nose buried in a book. He was a fortyish professional wearing a shirt and tie and a yarmulke. He invited me to sit down, and I slipped quickly into journalist mode.

I asked him to walk me through treatment. He said he used antipsychotic medications, similar to those I had taken, and talk therapy. He told a story about a typical patient: He had become anxious a few days after arriving in Jerusalem. Soon, he was washing his hands obsessively, and later bathing in public fountains. Eventually, the man completely lost touch with reality, stripped his hotel bed of its sheets, donned them like robes, and stood on a street corner proclaiming himself the Son of God. Emergency services took him to the hospital.

After an hour, Lichtenberg looked at his watch. "I have to be in a conference call in five minutes. Do you have any other questions?"

"Has a messiah ever said anything wise to you? Anything that would indicate that they might be the real thing?"

"Definitely," he said. "I find these patients fascinating and full of wisdom. Are there some who say brilliant and wise things and say something about what it means to be a human? One hundred percent. They teach me that all we have is our subjective experience. While they're here, being a messiah is what their experience is. And who am I to say it's pathological or wrong? For most, this is a temporary condition, and my goal is to help them recover the person they have been most of their lives and return them to their families. But while they are here? I treat them like they are the Messiah."

I found myself putting my hand on my heart when he said this. I was moved. I felt compassion for the messiahs, and I admired this doctor for his work. I also felt a new sense of compassion toward myself. I had been categorized, pathologized, put into so many boxes. I had been called unbalanced so often that I no longer wanted to live under the label of being mentally ill. I wanted to heal; I tried to heal. If I understood this man correctly, all my experiences, the easy ones, the exciting ones, the difficult ones, were legitimate.

Those labels had never defined me, although I thought they did. As soon as I was diagnosed as bipolar, I treated myself as sick. I bought into my own pathology. I was no longer human; I was only a patient. I told people I was sick. And that's how friends and family treated me. Like I was crazy. Now, sitting here on this afternoon with the light shining through the windows talking to this wise, kind man, I regretted all of it.

Lichtenberg's words eased my mind. Everybody's experience is legitimate. You might be a scientist who thinks the world is reducible to material things, and more power to you. That's your subjective experience. You might be a spiritual person, see everything in terms of energy or angels, and go for it. That's your experience. Nobody—no doctor, lawyer, or expert on anything—can tell you anything about who you are and what your background is, or whether it's healthy or unhealthy, legitimate or otherwise. As William James wrote in *The Varieties of Religious Experience*:

> Our normal waking consciousness, rational consciousness as we call it, is but one special type of consciousness, whilst all about it, parted from it by the filmiest of screens, there lie potential forms of consciousness entirely different. We may go through life without suspecting their existence; but apply the requisite stimulus, and at a touch they are there in all their completeness, definite types of mentality which probably somewhere have their field of application and adaptation. No account of the universe in its to-

tality can be final which leaves these other forms of consciousness quite disregarded.

Of course, the insurance companies need to use diagnoses to check the boxes and pay the bills, but to me, it felt like a game. My brother, David, who worked in the insurance business, embraced my diagnosis as much as I had. I guess he needed to view me as sick as badly as I did, even occasionally sharing my letters home with a psychiatrist he worked with. This felt like a massive betrayal, one that still stings to this day.

I thanked Dr. Lichtenberg, and as I got up and we shook hands, I said, "One more question, doctor. You said Jerusalem syndrome occurs on a spectrum. You see the severe cases. What do mild cases look like?"

"A mild case can present as a fascination or obsession with Jerusalem."

"I might have a case of Jerusalem syndrome?"

He didn't answer me. "Jerusalem syndrome can also present as an obsession that Jerusalem has the power to change us, to heal us. Brad, maybe it can."

I nodded in agreement. "Maybe it can," I repeated.

I left Lichtenberg's office and caught a cab to the Old City for one last spin around the sacred sites. It was sundown, and the famously dazzling Jerusalem light was layered with dusky shadows. I entered through the gate I had first entered the previous March: Damascus Gate.

When I moved through the cave-like opening, I found myself in a crowd of people fighting for shoulder room. As I made my way, once again, toward the Via Dolorosa, I felt a tug on my shirt and looked down to see a Palestinian boy who looked to be about ten or eleven with his hand out. He had a roundish face and a bowl haircut. He wore jeans and a white T-shirt, his short sleeves rolled up like a tough guy in a movie. He explained that he wanted to take me to the roof of his family's house to show me the view of the Dome of the Rock and all of Jerusalem—for ten shekels. I paid him, and he led me up a dark stairwell and through a door, and we emerged to stand on the tar-paper roof.

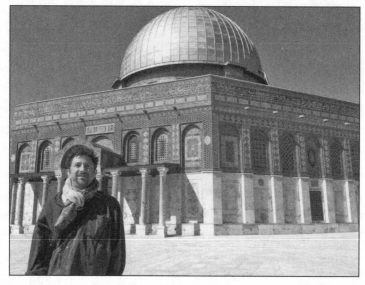

In February 2012, I asked a stranger to snap this picture of me in front of the Dome of the Rock in Jerusalem.

The view was astoundingly beautiful, raw and soul-stirring. The sun was setting over the Mount of Olives. Jerusalem spread out across the horizon. Laser-like beams of bright white light, as if emanating from heaven, were overlayed on a soft golden sea of orange to the west. The Dome of the Rock sparkled. We watched the sunset; I felt a sweet ecstasy fill up the core of my belly and rise into my chest. I felt like I did when I was sixteen, standing in front of the mirror pretending to be Dean Moriarty. I thanked him and then descended the stairs. Once again on street level, I took a right off Via Dolorosa and headed again toward the Church of the Holy Sepulchre. I didn't imagine I'd be back here any time soon. I had too much work on my life to do. And I wanted to see the crack in Adam's Chapel again. I wanted to know if it had any new messages for me.

I pulled open the heavy wooden door and entered the central nave, lit by candles. I walked to Adam's Chapel and stood, once again, before the crack that ran from ceiling to floor, from the site of Jesus's crucifixion to the site of Adam's tomb.

I searched my brain, my heart, my whole body for answers. Christians believe the crack was a sign that Jesus was God. Proof of his potency. But it didn't matter what it meant to somebody else. What did it mean to me?

I didn't think the answer so much as I felt it. I stared and stared, and I felt a wave of complex, deep emotion. It felt like everything, like when you follow a hard feeling such as anger, sadness, joy, elation . . . and you follow it to its end, to the tip of its tail, and the feeling changes slowly. It softens into . . . what? Bittersweetness. The feeling of It All. The feeling of every feeling when you take the time to pay attention and see the world as it might really be. Beautiful and broken. And then I looked around and noticed I was alone. Aren't we all always alone? No, we need each other. We need family, community, we need human touch. But aren't we always stuck in our heads, and really, underneath it all, running from the truth that nobody can do anything for us and that we must make sense of our time here the best we can on our own? Don't we all enter the world alone and leave it alone? Or is this just how I feel? I began to cry. My heart felt broken, as cracked as that line that split the world in two, thousands of years ago. And while that sounds negative, it felt like the opposite. I cried and felt grateful that I was finally in touch with my pain—I could feel it, in all its terrible truth.

I reasoned that if I could feel these emotions deeply, I could stop wondering, *Why me?* I could stop blaming others for my struggles. I could stop trying to figure out why it happened. And I could begin, finally, to *live*. I could relax. I could stop living in hypervigilance, waiting for the next person to hurt me. I could finally live with meaning and purpose and *feel everything*.

What if I could see my suffering as a gift that had broken me open and set my heart on this pilgrimage? If I saw my life as a pilgrimage of the heart, I sensed I might experience belonging, safety, abundance, even joy. What about peace? That too. All the states of feeling that were absent from my childhood. It was a seed that gave birth to my spiritual healing and awakening. My life wasn't a problem to be solved but a gift to be opened. The pain was real, but so was the resilience of my spirit.

I resolved to continue this pilgrimage of healing in the name of love. Love for myself, friends, the children of the world. I was ready to leave the dance of brokenness, blame, and oblivion. Being hurt didn't mean I was broken or needed to be fixed. I also knew that, over these years, I had created a secret theology that was designed to avoid any kind of hurt and prevent further suffering. It was time to become—and be—human again. No more pathology. As Teilhard de Chardin wrote, "To suffer is human. Tears are already in everything."

At the airport, when I told the security guard that I'd been in Palestine, he bombarded me with questions and then pointed to a room. I followed the instructions to take everything out of my bags and spread it out on the floor. My laptop was quickly confiscated. I felt deep sadness as I sat on the ground, stuffing my things back into my backpack after I was cleared to travel home. Heartbroken to be leaving this remarkable, religiously significant land, sorry to be ending this adventure and leaving the friends I'd made. I was leaving these real, meaningful experiences and turning them into memories. There was sadness in that too, but also opportunity.

I see now that my sorrow was also related to this fact: I needed to let go of some things. The Jesus story was about sacrifice. Ego death. What did it mean for me? I understood that I needed to stop chasing messiahs. I had to stop pathologizing myself. I had to be human. I had grown up with my family's ideas of right and wrong. I'd been taught that loyalty, more than any other quality, including love, was the essential thing in a relationship. Loyalty and perfection. Control. I had left childhood without much trust in myself. I trusted friends and relatives who might have helped me too little, and I trusted outright strangers, too much.

I understood that I needed to trust in myself in order to build a life I wanted to live. To create something and stick with it to the end. In this new digital world, with writing no longer a viable way to make a living, I'd need to get creative to make a decent living that made me proud. I couldn't imagine working for a corporation. I wanted to use the lessons I'd learned as a freelancer and create a business. Maybe an online business helping people write.

I didn't know what I would do with my experiences in the Holy Land, but I knew that I would not and could not return to the Christian faith. I couldn't ever again be "on fire" for Jesus.

But perhaps most important, I was ready to face the consequences of my self-betrayal. I had taken the drugs to disappear. I did it. I had continued to engage with my toxic family; I had believed their pathologizing of me and pathologized myself as well. Every day I worried that I was this or that diagnosis. The truth: I was human, which meant I was flawed *and* divine. I could hurt people. I could elevate and love people. As the plane took off over the Holy Land, I looked through the tiny fishbowl window at the beach below me. I drew a line in the sand for my self-abuse.

There was just one problem with the timing of this lurch toward self-care and self-love—as if we can ever control timing. Back home, my mother's cancer was advancing. Instead of facing my self-betrayal, I would need to face my mother's death. I wasn't ready for it. Is anyone ever?

seventeen

DOOR OF FAITH

Returning from Palestine ended one phase of my journey and began another. I settled back into my sad little studio apartment on Santa Fe's semirural west side. I sat in my one Ikea chair and peered past the gray walls through the one window at the leafy cottonwood tree in my landlord's elaborately xeriscaped backyard. I got up only to make PBJ sandwiches and coffee on the two hot plates that served as my stove. As pathetic as the situation might seem, I enjoyed the quiet. It felt good to be back home with two feet on the ground instead of running to catch planes, trains, and donkey carts. But the quiet came with a disturbing realization. My body was not liking the absence of the high doses of medications. Though I'd reduced the doses by only a third or so, I was experiencing withdrawal symptoms. Thankfully, I never had to deal with opiate withdrawals. I can only imagine. But I'd experienced withdrawal symptoms from psych meds before. Trust me, the pharmaceutical companies don't tell you this, but the drugs they develop in their laboratories are as addictive as anything you can buy on the street. Many of them, even basic antidepressants, can take weeks if not months of slow titration. I've felt the crazed panic when my drug-craving nervous system told me (falsely) that my windpipe was closing up. I've spent weeks with my field of vision interrupted by imaginary, insanity-inducing flashes of white lightning, and—the most brutal, for me, at least—the feeling of bugs, thousands of creeping, crawling insects, inside my legs when I try to sleep. I guess I'd been too busy and distracted to notice the onset of these symptoms, or maybe they just started. But now that I was home and I was reducing the medications further, the withdrawal symptoms felt intense and crazymaking. I couldn't even take a fifteen-minute nap without the bugs filling my legs with their intolerable creepy tickling.

I kicked. I paced back and forth. I went outside and walked the streets near my home. I scrounged in my bathroom vanity for old pill bottles that might contain some residue. I yanked underwear out of my top dresser drawer hoping to find a stray joint that I might have stashed a few years earlier after a camping trip. Nothing. I don't drink, for obvious reasons, or I'd have run to the nearest bar and downed a bottle of tequila. Nothing I did brought relief. Certainly, I didn't expect poetry to help, but I found myself sitting up, drinking herbal tea and reading Rumi.

You wouldn't think that adventure writing had much in common with mystical Sufi poetry. But today I understand that these two distinct genres have at least two things in common: One, the narrator longs to be somewhere that he's not. The mountain climbers in 1996 wanted off Mount Everest; Rumi longs to be closer to God. And two, there are obstacles in the way that must be overcome, including obstacles we humans create for ourselves, our own stubborn, fallible humanness.

Burning with longing fire.
Wanting to sleep with my head on your doorsill.
My living is composed only of trying to live in your
*   presence . . .*
I have lived on the lip of insanity, wanting to know rea-
*   sons, knocking on your door.*
It opens.
I've been knocking on the inside.

The last three lines slayed me. For the past decade, I had been wandering the world with my backpack full of pills seeking answers to life's big questions and trying to solve the problems of my life, which felt even bigger. But every time I took flight, hopped a train, or rode in a donkey cart, was I really, on some real but mystical level, doing something else? Was I knocking on the door from the inside? Was I already there?

Life has taken me on an extraordinary ride. I've had the opportunity to travel to many places that most people will never see: Greenland's Icecap; the long, cold halls of Star City, home to the Russian Space Agency; flower-decorated memorials to Palestinian suicide bombers; Varanasi's smoky burning ghat and the caves of Arunachala; remote Indian camps in the Amazon. I loved these places and my experiences in them. Adventurous travel was how I made my living during the first half of my life.

I thought adventure writing was my path. I thought maybe I'd discover myself, too, out there in the world. But I always failed, and I grew tired of that. I grew even more tired of who I found myself to be when I arrived back home. And by now you hopefully understand that disappearing into a fog of drugs was not my doctor's fault. It was mine. I stopped being able to face myself. I had no tools to calm my increasingly ragged nervous system. I could never have used the sawed-off shotgun either. I was too much of a coward. For me, using pills to disappear was as close to suicide as I could get. When that didn't work, in despair, feeling orphaned, from both my family and myself, I sought Jesus. Not in my heart, like most people; I tried to find him in the desert of a war-torn country where he had supposedly lived. And again, I failed to find myself out there.

Today I understand better. Life has two landscapes, external and internal. In the external landscape, we adventure through space, matter, and time. That's called life. But the internal journey is a solo expedition. If we want to find ourselves, we must adventure inward. What do we find here? Our hearts and the present moment. When we bring the adventure inside, we discover that the path to healing was here the entire time. It might seem like a cliché until you experience it for yourself. You and all you seek—maybe even God—are here now.

By the fall of 2012, I'd been in Santa Fe for eighteen years. I'd been through a lot of changes, from arriving there with my grad school sweetheart and a caravan of *Outside* colleagues, to leaving the magazine to live my dream as an adventure writer, to sitting in editorial meetings with JFK Jr. at *George* magazine's headquarters, to the total collapse of myself, to Paul's suicide. As the days grew shorter and the shadows grew longer, I wasn't sure whether I fit in Santa Fe anymore. But where would I go? I didn't have enough money to rent a U-Haul and fill it with gas. I had spent my last savings in the Holy Land.

And I still couldn't comprehend what happened there. I knew it would take months, maybe years, to gain perspective. I didn't rediscover faith in Jesus, and the quest had left me exasperated, exhausted by the seeking. I felt weary, as if I'd been seeking my entire life, maybe lifetimes. I felt weary, the way I suspect an old man feels after dragging around his soon-to-be corpse for seventy-five or eighty years. My arms and legs felt heavy. My heart was heavy.

I was also dealing with drug-induced brain fog. It was all consuming. I wasn't trying to peer through it; I was the fog. I embodied it. But was the hazy stupor caused solely by the medications? I suddenly had doubts. I was no longer taking Risperdal, and I'd reduced the dose of the other meds by half. Shouldn't the confusion be lifting? Instead of having a telescope for seeing the stars and a microscope for seeing at a cellular level, it felt like I was using them in reverse: I used the telescope for the cells and saw blur, and I used the microscope for the stars and saw blackness. As a result, I saw only confusion no matter where I looked.

The practical effect was that I struggled to make dinner plans, let alone a life plan. I was passive. And while I could discern a path leading through the jungle of my life to a light on the hill, I was overwhelmed by its chaotic zigs and zags, and I doubted I had the tools, the life skills, to make the journey to the light.

And yet the heaviness in my arms and legs and heart felt good: it felt like solid ground, like a remnant of the sorrow I'd felt at the crack. The heartbreak felt like maybe it was the way forward. I remembered the lines from the book of Thomas and remained convinced that they contained something for me: "If you bring forth what is within you, what you bring forth will save you. If you do not bring forth what is within you, what you do not bring forth will destroy you." But what was inside me that needed to come out? Was all this shifting inside my body something that wanted to come out?

I needed a break from Jesus, from all this self-interrogation. At a used bookstore, I picked up a copy of *The Wayfinders*, by Wade Davis, a writer I'd spoken to a few times when I worked at *Outside*. A Canadian cultural anthropologist, ethnobotanist, author, and photographer, Davis was an adventure writer on steroids, a man with a massive cerebral cortex. As a twentysomething editor, I'd grilled him on the phone about his experiences researching zombies in Haiti, which grew into the book and movie, *The Serpent and the Rainbow*. I felt deep admiration for Davis. His brain had astounding breadth and depth, and he embraced mythology and the unconscious, too.

The Wayfinders is a collection of lectures about his experiences with different cultures and how they cultivate and pass on what might be called wisdom. He attempts to understand what wisdom is and how it is similar and different across cultures and time. He describes a 1999 voyage on which Nainoa Thompson and members of the Polynesian Voyaging Society sailed a sixty-two-foot double-hulled canoe called the *Hokulea'a* twenty thousand kilometers from Hawaii to Rapa Nui, Easter Island, a target just twenty-three kilometers across. Thompson's navigational skills, learned from a Polynesian elder named Mau Piailug, consisted of the fundamental elements of the Polynesian world: wind, waves, clouds, stars, sun, moon, birds, fish, the water itself plus the wisdom he carried in his body and heart.

At one point, close to their goal, Nainoa snapped awake in a daze and realized that with the overcast skies and the sea fog, he had no idea where they were. He had lost the continuity of mind and memory essential to survival at sea. He masked his fear from the crew and in despair remembered Mau's words. Can you see the image of the island in your mind? He became calm and realized that he had already found the island. It was the *Hokulea'a*, and he had everything he needed on board the sacred canoe. Suddenly, the sky brightened, and a beam of warm light appeared on his shoulder. The clouds cleared and he followed that beam directly to the island of Rapa Nui.

I set down the book and placed my hand on my heart. I felt the heaviness in my body and thought about Jesus saying, "Bring out what is inside you, or it will kill you." If Thompson had lost track of his knowledge, if he had not brought it out, he might have killed himself and his crew. Maybe my grief needed to come out . . . and maybe so did my wisdom. Could I pull my future, a road map of healing, out of the sea like Thompson had with Easter Island? Could I pull a sense of having a full, unfragmented self out of the fog of my life? Could I pull out what was inside me and live, as Jesus said? Could I once again live a thriving, full, happy life? I wanted this more than you can ever know.

I hadn't called my parents since returning from Palestine. I often felt ambivalence about calling home. A longing for real connection, for family like some of my friends seemed to have, and fear of the disappointment and sadness I'd feel after performing the duty without feeling real love. Part of it was a lifetime of awkward conversations that never felt very emotionally connective. Part of it was not wanting to be judged for trying to pull my life together by hitting the road in the Holy Land. And, this time, part of it was my mom's illness.

Five years earlier, an ophthalmologist had discovered a tumor during a routine eye exam—ocular melanoma. She had her eye removed and replaced with a prosthetic. Then, she was told there was a fifty-fifty chance the cancer would return, this time in her liver. The last time I spoke to her was in July, and she sounded tired. She would never admit to me how bad the cancer was, and so I had to lean on my intuition and my own research. I knew from reading about ocular melanoma that hardly anybody survives longer than two or three years, even with the most advanced therapies, which she'd had.

"Hi, Mom, I'm back from Palestine. How are you doing?"

As soon as she spoke, I could feel that her battle with melanoma, which had metastasized to her liver and everywhere else, was nearing the end. Her nonchalant voice reminded me of the home environment I'd soon return to.

"Oh, I'm doing fine," she said.

I felt my diaphragm and intercostal muscles contract. "Really, Mom, how are you doing?"

"I guess I'm fine. Are you home for now? You aren't traveling anywhere soon, are you? What are you using for money?"

"I used the $3,500 from Uncle Wallace's estate sale that you sent me."

"I thought you'd save that. Or buy groceries with it."

"No, Uncle Wallace paid for my trip to Palestine. But *Newsweek* is going to run my travel article. So I'll break even." This was true.

We chatted for a few minutes about her garden, her church, her friends. And then I told her I loved her, and we said goodbye. As I hit End I felt sad. I was grateful for the opportunity to talk with her, but the conversation was achingly familiar and superficial. How I wished we could connect more deeply. Or, at least, have honest, real conversations that represented reality, about both good times and hard times.

I perked up by convincing myself that a drive to the countryside was what I needed. I would drive my truck to Abiquiu and visit the Christ in the Desert Monastery, located at the end of a twelve-mile dirt and gravel road at the foot of a red cliff beside the Chama River. I loved walking the grounds there and sitting next to the river. And by the time I returned home in the evening, hopefully my heartburn or whatever was going on in my chest would be gone.

I got in my truck and drove north on Highway 285/84, past Española to the Chama River valley. I passed Bo's gas station and the turnoff to Ghost Ranch, Georgia O'Keeffe's onetime home. I kept driving north. I disappeared into the piñon-freckled dreamscape of striated red cliffs and puffy white clouds against the bright sapphire sky. I continued to feel an ache in my heart and continued to dismiss it as my breakfast disagreeing with my stomach.

This magical land, featuring old, rusty Buicks on concrete blocks in front of small, adobe farmhouses and the occasional ladder flying across the sky, lifted by strong, westward winds, appears endless, timeless. For as long as I'd lived in Santa Fe, I was drawn to this region, immortalized in the abstract expressionism of Georgia O'Keeffe. About ten miles north of Abiquiu, I turned left onto Forest Road 151 and headed west in the direction of Christ in the Desert, a gathering of quaint adobe structures that's home to a community of Benedictine monks called to be in silent communion with their God.

Finding a bench that faced the quiet hillside surrounding the monastery, I rested my hand on my heart and did nothing else. I felt the ache, a beautiful, painful, soulful ache. I thought of my mother and our conversation. I so wished we could get real with each other. In my family, everything was always *fine*, and it seemed to be more so when things weren't actually fine at all. So northern European of us. And then I thought about the crack in the Holy Sepulchre and the Mount of Olives, and all those intense emotions that fueled my two five-week pilgrimages. Could I simply steep in these beautiful memories rather than trying to make sense of them? I craved that my past would resolve into my soul and become part of me. Was that why my heart ached?

If Jesus was about anything, his message was about the heart. Not the limited view of the heart as the organ that pumps blood but the heart of poets and increasingly, science, too. Science is catching up to what poets have always known. New research shows that the area around the heart contains millions of neurons similar to those found in the brain. Its electrical current is fifty to sixty times stronger than that of the brain. Its electromagnetic current is five thousand times stronger. The presence of these neurons suggests that the heart is a center of intelligence. The electromagnetic current says it sends and receives signals far outside the body. The heart creates a field of energy, one more powerful than our thinking brains.

I got up from the bench and headed back toward the highway. As the road climbed and I gazed out across the Chama River valley, I had an idea. I turned off the road and parked near a boat takeout. Nobody was around. I took my clothes off and waded into a rounded-out river bend known as Big Eddy. In September, the river runs shallow, and the Class III rapids are gone, replaced by a gentle rippling current. I swam out to the middle of Big Eddy, and there I bobbed, floated, and swam. The water, snowmelt from the high Rockies to the north, felt like ice against my skin. My muscles relaxed, as if giving up on my unconscious habit of trying against all reason to hold the universe together. And then I felt my mind give up on holding the universe together, too. What a relief. *Why don't I come here more often, like every damn day?* The submerged log in Arkansas that nearly killed me was a thousand miles away, literally, and it was nowhere to be found in my mind, either. My father, my entire family, was absent too. I swam for thirty or forty minutes, and then I tiptoed back to the sandy bank to towel off with an extra sweater I found on the back seat. I gathered sticks and grabbed a few pieces of firewood I'd brought from town. I lit a campfire inside a rock ring that a stranger before me had built. The sun was setting over the cliffs across the river. I stared into the fire, listening to the hypnotic music of water tumbling between two banks and carving deeper into the earth. A short time later, the evening stars of Mars, Jupiter, and Venus glowed brightly in the sky. I leaned back and rested my head on the sun-warmed sand. I gazed up at the Milky Way; it looked as if God had tipped over a bottle, spilling billions upon billions of gallons of the stuff.

I took a massive breath that seemed to find its way to my toes. I relaxed my shoulders, which had been hugging my skull like earmuffs. I felt like I was home, if only momentarily. My mind was quiet except for these words, which rose from my heart and tumbled out my mouth and washed over my body. My heart seemed to tell me to let go of the seeking. Maybe I needed to let go of a whole hell of a lot more. Things I wasn't aware that I was clinging too tightly to.

Let it all go, man. Let it all go, man. Just, let it all go, man. Let it all go. Let it all go, man. Let it all go—down this river and on to the Gulf of Mexico.

I put out the fire and drove back to Santa Fe. Over the next weeks, I tried to get real with myself, practical. *How can I make a living with the skills I have?* I can edit and I can write. Stop with the selling junk. That is never going to work. How had I ever thought that would work? I hired a friend to build a personal website. I included a bio and listed all the articles I'd written. I added a page offering to coach and edit for people who wanted to write about travel. I thought about moving to someplace new, too. But where?

I thought about my family and Bob Dylan, a childhood hero. He left his home state of Minnesota at age twenty and never looked back. In this youthful and rebellious act, he seemed to obliterate his past and claim a new, bold future in service only to the man he felt and knew himself to be. For me, age twenty was many moons ago, but maybe I needed to connect with my inner Bob to do that now. Maybe my family felt ambivalent about me too. Wouldn't we all be better off if I just walked away and never looked back?

eighteen

STOP CHASING!

W HEN DI AND I WERE STILL MARRIED, OUR FRIENDS ANDREW and Madeleine took us to a small concert given by Krishna Das at Santa Fe's Unitarian Universalist Church. Despite my grumpy journalist misgivings about the whole thing, I was mesmerized by his spare music. My chest cavity vibrated like a cello. Between songs, Krishna Das told stories about his time in India. He offered a deep, embodied wisdom in a thick New York accent with smatterings of profanity and humble smiles. He explained that singing the names of god was his spiritual practice. His way of meditating. He said that he was singing to Maharaj-ji, his guru. Even though Maharaj-ji had left his body, Krishna Das believed that his guru now existed everywhere. As he wrote in his book

> Maharaji didn't do much teaching. He never wrote books. When we asked him how do we become enlightened, he said, serve people, feed people. Love everyone, serve everyone, remember God. Chanting pulls me out of my own bullshit and brings me back to the present moment, back to myself. As time goes on, I've seen changes in my life for the better. I have noticed that I spend less and less time in negative states of mind. I don't judge myself so harshly. I become less and less involved with thinking about myself so much. I've become more open and at ease with myself and what comes to me in life. And all this from singing the names of God.

The concert happened ten years before my Holy Land wanderings. At the time, I considered myself agnostic, bordering on atheist. But I did enjoy the singing, and I felt curious about this man and his wild stories. I had a sense that something about him was trustworthy. It didn't make a stitch of sense to my science-oriented, journalistic mind, but somehow it made perfect sense to the part of me that had always been interested in spiritual matters and had mystical experiences. I really didn't know what to make of the mystical aspects of the practice Krishna Das described in such passionate detail. Which part of myself should I trust and seek to be in alignment with? The fact-based journalist atheist? Or the spiritual Brad who was open to the wild, weird possibilities that life seemed to also offer?

I enjoyed the night enough that I googled Krishna Das when I got home. Krishna Das was born Jeffrey Kagel to a Jewish family on Long Island. He grew up playing sports and feeling depressed, and I could read between the lines that his own family was dysfunctional. During college, he discovered LSD, and, like so many people in the 1960s, he was changed by the expanded view of himself and the world brought on by the drug. Ultimately, LSD could not shake his depression. In fact, he said in an interview I read, it likely made the feelings of despair even worse. During this period, he moved to a farm in Pennsylvania, where he lived alone. His life began to change for the better when he met Ram Dass.

I opened a new browser window and googled Ram Dass. I skimmed over what I already knew about his life as Richard Alpert, the Harvard expert in Western psychology and human personality who famously conducted LSD research with Timothy Leary.

In 1967, Alpert took LSD to India, hoping to see what sense India's famous holy men could make of the drug. Was it a tool that could aid in expanding consciousness? Was it a spiritual substance? He didn't learn much from India's saints. But in Kathmandu, he met a long-haired, bearded, six-foot-seven California surfer who'd been living as a wandering ascetic in India for four years. Bhagavan Das had grown up Kermit Michael Riggs and was traveling around India, living with swamis, *sadhus*, Buddhist monks, and gurus. They struck up a conversation, and Bhagavan Das mentioned that he was going to see his guru in the Himalayan foothills of northern India. Alpert begged to go with him. They climbed into Alpert's jeep, and off they went for the village of Kainchi, site of a temple to Hanuman and the summer home of an Indian holy man named Neem Karoli Baba, who went by Maharaj-ji. They found him with a group of disciples on a hillside near the former British hill station of Nainital. Alpert followed Bhagavan Das up the hill, and then, as Alpert approached, he was suddenly filled with intense emotion. *Love.* This nebbish professor of psychology dropped to his hands and knees and touched Maharaj-ji's feet. He wept. Later, Maharaj-ji rocked Alpert's inner world when he told him that he knew what he was thinking the previous night. He'd taken a walk and thought about his mother, who died the previous year. Maharaj-ji even knew that his mother's illness involved her spleen.

The rest of this story is well known in contemporary US spiritual circles. Alpert became a devotee of Neem Karoli Baba. He spent a year living at or near his guru's small ashram in Kainchi. Maharaj-ji gave him a new spiritual name, Ram Dass, Servant of Ram, the avatar of Vishnu, the Hindu god who sustains and preserves the universe. Yes, Ram Dass gave his guru enough LSD "to send a horse to the moon," and it had no effect on him. Later, after he returned to the United States, Ram Dass wore the white clothes of a holy man and began lecturing to audiences about yoga and the essential teachings of his guru. He wrote a strange, hand-printed best-selling book called *Be Here Now* that remains a spiritual classic. Ram Dass suffered a debilitating stroke in 1997 at age sixty-six and spent the next twenty-two years in a wheelchair suffering from partial paralysis and difficulty speaking. He died in 2019.

I realized I had seen Ram Dass speak in the early 2000s, around the time I began my descent into the numbness of strong antipsychotic medications, but I barely remembered the talk. Soon afterward, I met Janis, an eccentric and witchy—in a good way—friend of Andrea's who struggled with mental health issues and occasional homelessness. She sometimes stayed with us in the spare bedroom. One day, she plopped her ancient copy of *Be Here Now* down on the desk in my office. I picked it up and turned a few pages. It was from the hippie era. It was printed on yellow paper and had odd, handwritten lettering—like something self-published by a sorcerer. I read the introduction but could make no sense of the nonlinear writing and the far-out thoughts.

But now, years later, the thread of Ram Dass and the thread of Krishna Das began to swirl together inside me. I was doing a lot of reading. Perhaps I was searching for my next Bible. My next Jesus. After all I'd been through in my life, I was tired of psychology. Psychiatry had seduced me and then brutalized and pathologized me. I was weary of the rat race, too. I was doubtful that achievement mattered a whit in the big scheme of things. I was ready to leave the American Dream and all the chasing of money, status, and personal identity behind. I was ready for love, too. Call it hippie-dippie bullshit, but I wanted it in my life. I wanted it more than anything. I didn't care that it might seem quaint and dated to my friends and colleagues from my journalism days.

I found Ram Dass's story of personal transformation—from neurotic Harvard intellectual to deeply emotional and spiritual being—to be more than inspirational. Why? Because of how dramatic and rebellious the transformation was. As a Harvard psychology professor, he knew practically everything there is to know about human personality and psychology. He had developed status and wealth based on his intellect. But his guru taught him to see that none of that mattered, and maybe Western psychology wasn't a very accurate or useful way to think about human beings. Maharaj-ji taught him that there were spiritual realms more "real" than physical reality. But more than that, Maharaj-ji taught him that the only thing that mattered was love. Maharaj-ji didn't merely teach Ram Dass this. He showed him. According to many disciples of Neem Karoli Baba, the Himalayan guru loved you from the inside out. And he challenged Ram Dass to face his anger. Maharaj-ji's teachings could be boiled down to two commandments: "Love everyone and tell the truth." Period. Maharaj-ji taught that, at the root, we are love.

Ram Dass didn't merely sacrifice money and status. He abandoned his entire egoic identity as a successful, highly paid intellectual and became a spiritual teacher, discussing matters of the heart that he'd learned from his Indian guru. In other words, Ram Dass gave up power. This is not what a man in America does. And this fascinated me. It fired me up.

In Ram Dass, I saw a possible road map for my own healing. I started listening to every recording I could find of him delivering spiritual teachings. While some of his fans saw him as an enlightened being in those first years after his time with Maharaj-ji, I experienced him differently. Even after he'd abandoned his professorial identity for that of a holy man, I could still hear in his voice his neurosis and anger. Despite the dominant narrative about Ram Dass, he struggled to find peace with himself his entire life. And guess what? He got there. Mostly. I believe this. Maybe I could too. Back when I first encountered him, I was cynical, closed-minded. But I wasn't the same person anymore. Ram Dass talked about the possibility that we can overcome our loneliness by tapping into God. I'd tried this, both as a kid and on my recent travels in the Holy Land. I was skeptical. But I certainly would love to find out it was true. I admit, gullibility and hopefulness haven't always served me in my life. But Ram Dass seemed to have faith in something. Maybe in his guru, maybe also in himself. But also in life. In the adventure of life. I wanted that too.

I started to fall asleep at night reading *Be Here Now* and listening to Krishna Das.

We take steps forward and we take steps back on this journey, don't we? One morning I felt more alone that I'd felt in a long time. I wondered what Andrea was doing. Was she sitting in her beautiful garden drinking coffee and admiring the flowers? It sounded lovely. I looked around at my gray apartment. She was a kind, beautiful woman. Complicated, too. But so was I. As I fell asleep, I wondered whether I'd made a poor decision when I told her I wanted to end the relationship. I had such confusion around my feelings. My heart, my desire, was so often at odds with my addled nervous system. I didn't know what inner messages to listen to.

At 2 a.m., I was still lying awake. I got out of bed and called her. She didn't answer. I drove over to her house. I knocked on her gate. But a man answered. "Go away. Andrea's busy."

Shit! She's moved on.

I spent the rest of the night at Dunkin' Donuts drinking coffee and reading. I couldn't sit at home alone. The next day, Andrea called me. She was gracious, but she said she had begun seeing a man she'd dated once before. I told her I missed her. I asked her whether we could meet to talk about reuniting. She was wary. I pleaded with her to see me. When I arrived at her house that evening, I suddenly felt convinced I'd screwed up in breaking up. I missed her. I missed her eccentric ways, her impractical house filled with nineteenth-century Russian and French antiques, even her stories about being the granddaughter of a Castilian princess. I missed the love we had, which had felt true and real when we lived together.

Andrea and I did reunite, and a few weeks later, we impulsively and unwisely married at the courthouse. I moved back into her magical mystery tour of a home. I felt totally filled up with love and, once again, infatuated with her.

Having a companion again gave me the strength I needed to call home to check on my mother. I knew she wasn't doing well. After we chatted, I bought two plane tickets from Albuquerque to Kansas City. Andrea and I checked in to a hotel and took a taxi to my parents' house. I hugged my mother, and I shook my father's hand. My mother, usually so hopeful and positive, looked tired. She used a walker to get around the house. She complained of the extreme pain in her shin bone where the cancer now was.

As we all sat down to dinner, I felt a little lurch of dread. My family had met Andrea before; they made it obvious that they didn't think highly of her. She suffered from trauma and depression and hadn't built a conventional career. Her empty bank account, combined with her love of talking about her aristocratic Russian family's colorful past, went over with my midwestern family like champagne at a funeral. As we sat around the dinner table, noshing on Kansas City beef barbecue, Andrea began a story about her family's close ties to the Romanovs. I knew her stories to be true, even if they might come across as outrageous and self-serving, as I'd spent hours flipping through photo albums of her family living in a mansion in Paris with the grandson of Czar Nicholas II after the Russian Revolution. Andrea, in turn, had to listen to my family's hagiographic stories about our Swedish heritage. Family pride is family pride. But my father, brother, and sister-in-law didn't see this. They interrogated her like trial lawyers, demanding that she present incontrovertible proof of her stories. My mother must have seen my anger, or perhaps she saw me looking at my father, trying to telepathically communicate to him to call off the wolves. The evening ended with Andrea in tears and me shaking with rage.

After dessert, Andrea retreated to our room, and my mother and I sat on the screened-in porch. Pain medicine had dulled her eyes and slurred her speech. I felt like I was with somebody other than the woman who'd given me life and raised me. A people pleaser like me, she seemed less hopeful. Hope, I think, had been her coping mechanism through my father's drinking and chronic cheating. She wasn't seeing the bright side of her cancer anymore. And therefore, she felt more real, more connected with the truth of how the world works. I held her hand.

"I'm sorry, Mom. I'm sorry you're going through this. What do you need from me?"

Suddenly, she shifted back to hope. "I'm going to be okay."

"Okay, Mom."

"Are you going to be okay?" she asked.

"Yes, I'm on a good path now. I know it might not seem like it, but I am."

Then she gave me a gift I could have used decades earlier, although I wouldn't be able to use it for another few years. I didn't know it then, but this would be our last private talk before she died. Her gift was three simple sentences, a command, a statement of irrefutable truth: "Stop chasing your father, Brad. Just stop. You will never get what you want from him."

My body felt the truth of what she was saying, but my mind rejected it. Though I would think about her words often, I wasn't ready to hear them. Not yet. Years later, when I told a therapist I was working with my mother's words, she paused the session and looked at me solemnly: "Can you hear that deeply? Can you feel that in your body? Death-bed statements like this tend to be things to pay deep attention to." I listened to my therapist with rapt attention, but, in that moment, I still couldn't feel the truth of what my mother had said. I still had too much hope that my father would change. I had too much hope that my family could change. I had too much hope that I could magically change my past and suddenly wake up with healthy childhood memories. I had too much hope that I could erase the years of lying on a couch, dissociated, depressed, and over-medicated. I had too much hope that I'd wake up and be somebody else.

Several weeks after Andrea and I returned home from that trip, I called my parents to check in. My father answered.

"How's she doing?"

"We are dealing with some kidney issues," he said. "But we have her on some new medicine for it."

I knew that wasn't a good sign.

"Her cancer has moved into her bones. She's hurting. But we have some new pain meds, too."

This sounded even worse.

"Okay, I'll book a flight."

His response felt awful to hear, but it didn't surprise me.

"That's not necessary, Brad."

"Um, it seems pretty clear that she's not doing very well. I'd like to spend some time with her while I still can."

My father pushed against that idea. "You are being dramatic. We have her symptoms under control."

"Her symptoms? She's dying, Dad."

"You're not a doctor, Brad. I'm in contact with the doctor every day. We have signed her up for a new drug trial. The doctor is hopeful about it."

"Bullshit." As soon as the word left my mouth, I dissolved into shame. I had disrespected my father. I softened my tone, and for the last minute of the phone call I became a people pleaser again.

I bought a plane ticket as soon as I hung up the phone. In the hospital, I found my mother delirious from a high dose of pain-controlling opioids. I sat on the bed and held her hand, and we talked. It was clear that she was close to the end. A quick conversation with the doctor in the hallway confirmed this. I read her a short passage from my Palestine travel essay in progress, and she asked me, "What was it really like there?" and "Why do you like going to those crazy places?"

As I looked up from the page, I knew in my body that these few minutes were the last time we would be together when she still was conscious. Even if my dad couldn't see that she was dying, I could. I didn't so much picture the forty-five years of my life as much as I felt them rising out of my muscle, bone, and organs. I felt in my liver the weird way that experiences fade into the past. I felt the way that we humans, even parents and children, come together for short periods of time and then fall away. I also felt that orphan feeling again. Yes, she was my mother. I knew she loved me. And I suddenly could accept something that I'd been in denial about: she had done her best. Maybe my father had, too. I don't know. There was no use in holding grudges or asking questions about why I never felt at home when I was with my family. There was no explanation. I had been born into this family, but we really didn't have much in common. I felt gratitude, too, for all the love she had given me.

In that moment, I also I remembered the oddest of things: Once, when I was a sophomore in college, she'd visited me at my apartment, and she took me out shopping for clothes. I suggested a secondhand store favored by downscale hipsters, and there she spotted a maroon beret sitting high on a shelf. I never would have considered buying it for myself. I never would have imagined wearing it or that my mother would consider purchasing it for me. She was a Macy's woman who favored me in Izod shirts and khaki slacks. She hated my beard. But on this day, she pointed at the beret.

"I want to get that for you," she said.

I looked up at this utterly impractical used maroon beret with a smile, inside and outside. I doubted I would wear it, but I thought I knew what was up with her. She was trying to show me that she saw my out-of-the-box, creative side. I let her buy the beret for me. I wore it a couple of times, and then I hung it on a floor lamp, where it stayed. But I still remember that day and that beret as the first time I felt seen, really seen, by either of my parents. I don't know where that beret is today. But every time I hear Prince's "Raspberry Beret," I smile.

The day after that hospital visit, a Monday, my mother returned to her big, beautiful house on the golf course to die in her own bedroom. She fell into a coma almost immediately. For four days and nights, we took turns sitting with her, as her breathing slowed to only six breaths per minute. During her last moments, I struggled to stay grounded and nonreactive and at the same time to try to feel the sadness. I was losing the woman who gave birth to me, who nursed me, and held me—but she was also the woman who colluded with my father. A crowd of my parents' church friends gathered in the bedroom with our family. With all eyes on him, my father doted over her. The man who used to walk ten paces ahead of her now kissed her dehydrated lips. I couldn't decide if his attentiveness was sweet or pure show business. And even having these thoughts felt disgusting to me. And that was part of the problem. I didn't know what was true about my family or me. I didn't know whether he really knew her. I didn't know whether any of us really knew each other. When I spoke up, she'd said nothing. She enabled the drinking and the lies, and although I knew that she had suffered greatly, she also failed me. She allowed the scapegoating to occur. And yet she was my mother.

Unhealed dysfunctional families do not weather crises well. I was determined to stay out of family arguments while also standing up for myself. I feared I wasn't up to the task. I feared that, when the sarcasm, sniping, and dictator-like top-down control that was the rule of law in my family emerged, I would lose my shit. It didn't help that my father seemed uncomfortable with me, and he seemed to need to chip away at my agency. He burst into the bedroom when I was visiting with Mom alone and scolded me for putting on some light acoustic music by artists that I knew she liked.

"Brad, listen, I determine what music is played in here, not you," he said. "Do not change the play list. I know what Mom wants to hear."

"Okay, Dad." I nodded and switched the music back to Susan Boyle from *America's Got Talent* singing, "I Dreamed a Dream."

One morning, my mom's brother Ken, with whom she was close, asked me to call him if she seemed to be fading so that he could be there at the end, but when I excused myself to call him to say she might be close, Lisa, my sister-in-law, grabbed the phone out of my hand, explaining angrily that my father was charge of the situation and that I had no right to call Ken.

I felt like throwing my hands up then. But again, I tried to remain grounded and helpful. Four days after she returned home, on December 7, 2012, my mother died. She tried to take one more breath, and, when she couldn't, one big teardrop, bigger than any tear I'd seen, fell from her prosthetic eye, the left one, where her cancer had first presented. She was seventy-three.

To be honest, I tried to feel the sadness, but I couldn't. When you live in hypervigilance, waiting for the next insult, you become hardwired against feeling anything. But a few minutes later, as I sat alone with her body and held her still-warm hand, I pressed my other hand into my own heart. I felt her. I felt me. I felt our almost fifty-year-long soul connection, if only for a few short moments. My mind tunneled back in time, through the sweet times and the difficult times: Mom standing in front of the microwave in her pink nightgown warming a cup of milk to give to me after I'd knocked on their bedroom door at two in the morning and told her I hadn't slept a wink—the third night of this insomnia. I remembered the confused, angry look on her face after I'd burned and blistered my face while playing with the gas grill. "Don't get mad at me now please, just help me," I said.

I remembered other times as well: sitting on the couch in the living room, my arms wrapped around her as she cried, asking whether I thought she should stay with my father or leave him. I held her tight. I knew what I wanted. And I knew that she wouldn't do it, that maybe she couldn't do it.

"Get out of this marriage," I said. "You deserve better. I know there's a man out there who will love you like you deserve."

In retrospect, I see a curious, sad pattern. I cared more that she would find a new man than that I would have a stable home situation. She was my mother, but I was parenting her. By age fifteen, I had been co-opted into codependent enmeshment in my relationships. After that first time I held her and comforted her, my chest hurt whenever I looked at her, which was every day. I lost the ability to see her as *my* parent, my protector, my rock in the stream to stand on.

I began worrying about her when I was at school. Was she happy or sad? Was my dad cheating on her again? Was he pissing the bed again? I lost the ability to feel myself or know what I wanted or needed. I felt so sorry for her. She seemed trapped. I knew that leaving a wealthy, high-status man would be hard for a woman who had set her own career aside to raise kids. I knew she enjoyed a luxurious lifestyle, and that this too would be difficult to leave behind. She never left. And I never blamed her for it.

Years later, in some ways, I am not as forgiving. She didn't do what was right. By staying with him, she allowed his chaos, drinking, and sarcastic put-downs to continue. I have no doubt that I left childhood more psychologically damaged than I would have been if she'd left. Life as a divorced mother in her financial position would have been difficult. I understood her decision even better after my father reaped a million-dollar financial windfall after the death of a key client. And then there was another financial bump after the deaths of his wealthy aunt and uncle. I have no idea how much he made from those estates, but their lifestyle instantly became far more luxurious. They moved to a four-thousand-square-foot home in a gated community on a golf course. They acquired multiple time-shares in Palm Desert and Arizona. My mother bought a fur coat. They drove Lincolns and Lexuses. They traveled all over the world. I remember talking to my mother on the car phone as they rode in a limousine to see Elton John. She sent a picture of them. They posed arm in arm, as Sir Elton played piano a short distance behind them. I guess she was happy. I assume they loved each other to the end, which I don't understand. I know relationships are hard, and there are gifts from sticking with it through difficult times. But on the eve of her death, I felt confused and bitter. I'm not proud of that feeling, but it's honest. Even as she died, as that big tear fell from her eye, I couldn't feel who I was or how I felt about her, or me, or the two of us, or anything.

After the private time with my mother's body, the family gathered in the bedroom for a prayer. Andrea spoke up, saying that she would be happy to stay with my mother's body while the nurses cleaned her to be taken to the mortuary. She told me later that her family always did this, to honor the dead so that they weren't with strangers in death. Her statement must have triggered something deep inside my brother. He moved toward her, his voice angry and his body threatening, and said, "You will *not* do anything of the sort! We are not Russians!" My brother is a lifelong athlete—fit and strong. I needed to say something in support of Andrea. So many times, nobody had stood up for me in my family dynamic when abusive language was employed.

"You will not speak to my wife so aggressively," I said.

He stepped toward me and thrust his finger into my chest. "Let's take this outside and finish this." His words felt like an invitation to solve this issue, and maybe all our issues, with physical violence. I backed away from him and left the room.

I left the house and walked through the streets of my parents' gated community. I felt angry, but I also felt tired of feeling angry. *What would Ram Dass tell me to do now?* He'd say, "Tell the truth, and lose the anger." I was good at being a truth teller, especially when I was naming the denial that fueled my family's false narrative, but I wasn't so good at losing the anger. In fact, I was a failure at anger. I tried to calm my nervous system, and I thought about how Andrea and I could get out of this place and back to Santa Fe. Unfortunately, we had a full week of funeral preparation ahead of us. I wanted to stay to honor my mother.

My mother's funeral drew four or five hundred people. All her service to the Junior League, the country club, the church, and her job as an educator for kids living with complicated disabilities paid off with a larger-than-life send-off. During the planning of the funeral, my father had asked who in our family wanted to say something. Both my brother and I raised our hands, but only my brother was allowed to speak. Later, my father said I could have the honor of editing the obituary my brother would write. I went easy, only adding the necessary commas after the names of cities and states. But when my brother and father examined my work, they reacted angrily, questioning not just the need for the commas but my two decades as a professional editor and my master's degree in journalism. "David, go ahead and take out all those weird commas," my father said. "I'm not sure Brad's right about them." By now, I was as amused as much as I was angry. And yes, this slight hurt. A comma marks a pause, gives space for a breath, nothing more. Adding a few commas was the smallest of contributions to the family's mourning of my mother's death. Adding commas was part of the job, the work I'd performed for a decade and a half. I was, if nothing else, a very good editor. Not only did they erase my breath, but they also dismissed and mocked it. I tried to smile. I might even have succeeded. But I was getting damn close to finally seeing the truth, and the commas brought me one step closer.

After the funeral, I stood alone, holding a plate of ham sandwiches and cookies, gazing out through the cold December air at the golf fairway and the haunting shadows of tree branches caught in the nearby streetlights, when my sister, who is a little more empathetic but also very loyal to the family's narrative of perfection, approached me. We were not close, but there was some kindness between us. I wondered what she was coming to say. I heard her voice while my back was turned. I tried to feel my feet against the wood floor. I tried to stay with the solidness of my organs. I was filled with hope for a pleasant, connective conversation but feared a put-down. Molly, like all of us kids, had learned the art of the put-down, and sometimes it seemed that the sarcasm and personal digs were the only way we had to connect. Sometimes a put-down was followed by an awkward half apology, but usually not. And any complaint was surely followed by a reminder, "Oh, come on, you're too sensitive."

"Brad . . ."

I turned around. "Hi, Molly."

And then she finished what she'd come to say: "You're so weird."

I know she was hurting; I knew everybody was hurting. I knew it didn't come from a hurtful place but from a hurt place. It was nothing that that she hadn't said to me before, but this time I heard it. In the past, I tried to let it roll off and told myself that it wasn't abusive, wasn't mean, and that, yeah, maybe I was a bit weird.

But now, at my mother's funeral, while I was lost in thoughtful re-flection and not in a family argument, I finally heard her. I came to a new understanding. Not even my commas were welcome in this family. It was so absurd, it was almost funny. They'd been telling me this for most of my life, I believe, and I had refused to hear it. Who wants to acknowl-edge that your own family doesn't love you? That they don't wish the best for you. That they see you as the source of their problems. Dysfunctional families spread the story that they would be better off without the family scapegoat. The family scapegoat is the perfect lowly beast to carry the burden of the family's uncomfortable projections. How easy would it be if that shadowy figure would just . . . disappear . . . and carry off all the problems with it. In the difficult days after my mother's funeral, if I had any doubt that I was the scapegoat, the garbage dump for their difficult feelings about themselves, that doubt was finally gone. I flew back to Santa Fe with a new awareness and a new plan to limit my involvement with my family.

To this day, my father and siblings seem to be content with the lie that it was perfect—except for me. We are all traumatized. I cannot speak to how it impacted other family members, but part of my life's work has been untangling my true self from the self that was created by family dynamics that are difficult.

After my mother's death, if I hoped for refuge in a replacement family, I wouldn't find it in my new marriage. Soon after we returned home from Kansas City, Andrea began saying she wanted to move to California. I didn't want that, and I told her, but she didn't seem to hear me. She began packing her belongings into boxes for the move. I told her again I wasn't moving to California. She kept packing. No, she didn't want a divorce, but yes, we were moving to California. That spring, I learned that she had been emailing and talking on the phone with a man in California. I wasn't sure if it was an emotional affair, but it seemed like it. I told her I was moving out and that I wanted a divorce. I knew in my body that I needed to leave her and I needed to leave Santa Fe. This small, creative city had served as my life raft for almost twenty years. I arrived here as an earnest twenty-eight-year-old journalist working hard to become a successful senior editor and writer. I felt hopeful about my future. I was madly in love with my grad school sweetheart. I was gung ho about the American Dream, too. But no more. The lashings that held that raft together were frayed and ready to pop. And I needed to act now, before I was flailing around in the floodwaters of life without a life raft. I wanted out. Of what? My own skin. My life. But this time, I didn't listen to my inner critic's hopeless rants. Now, I had something to lean on. I had found it while wandering in the Holy Land, and I brought it back with me. It was alive inside my body, in a place where nobody could steal it and where I couldn't overlook it. I'm talking about faith. I wasn't all alone twisting in the wind anymore. I had a companion, a mentor I could trust. I had faith. Faith in myself. And I was not going to abandon myself again.

Two months later, I packed my things into my Ford Ranger pickup. Without telling a soul, I drove to the edge of town and hopped onto I-25. I was done with Santa Fe. I was done with a lot of things. But I wasn't done with myself. I had already leased an apartment in Boulder,

Colorado, about six hours north. Why Boulder? I wanted to stay close to the Rocky Mountains. I felt grounded in the Rockies. I had visited Boulder only once, but I appreciated its progressive politics and was curious about its reputation as a spiritual center. Ram Dass and other highly regarded American spiritual teachers, including Jack Kornfield and poet Allen Ginsberg, had taught at Boulder's renowned Buddhist institute of higher learning, Naropa University. But to be honest, I chose Boulder on a hunch. On faith.

I had cued up *Door of Faith*, by Krishna Das, in the CD player. As the mud-colored houses and green brush of New Mexico transitioned to the more grandiose, glaciated peaks of Colorado, one song stood out to me, "Puja," an homage in Sanskrit, a spiritual offering to Shiva.

Here's one interpretation of the chant:

> *I bow to Lord Shiva, the Guru, the Self of All.*
> *Living with everything as its true nature. Supreme peace.*
> *Needing no support, but sustaining and supporting all.*
> *Illuminating the entire universe with the light of*
> *consciousness.*

I played it over and over, letting images of my 1999 travels in Varanasi swirl in my mind.

As the harmonium vibrated and Krishna Das moaned, I was back at the smoky burning ghat, watching the flames engulf the human body. I was inside the Shiva temple, in awe of the mumbling *sadhus* praying to Shiva, the Dark Lord, the god of destruction and rebirth. What is another name for the process of destruction and rebirth? Transformation. No longer was I thinking about being transformed. In that moment, I wasn't trying to analyze or plan my way into transformation. I was letting the music transform me.

I thought about the album's title: *Door of Faith*. Faith as a door. A door I could walk through? Confused about most of the Sanskrit words, I hummed along to that album for the next six hours as I drove past the turnoff to my favorite fly-fishing spot on the Pecos River, past Hermits Peak, where I had camped often with my *Outside* colleagues, past the barren flat desert near Wagon Mound and the soulless fast-food joints of Raton. I knew what needed to happen next in my life. I was going to Boulder, and I was going to stop chasing Jesus, doctors, and my father. I was going to save myself. Because I finally understood a truth I probably should have learned four decades earlier, a truth most people learn when they first leave home: nobody was coming for me. Nobody was going to pick me out of the crowd and make me the man I wanted to be. It was up to me.

I pondered the only kind of faith I'd known about growing up: Christian faith. It's not an easy concept, though the word is thrown around every Sunday in churches and on Christian TV and radio shows. For me, faith is not synonymous with belief. Belief implies agreement with facts, and in fact Søren Kierkegaard coined the term "leap of faith" to describe the way Christian faith requires one to disavow seeing facts as facts. For me, faith is similar to the Sanskrit word *shraddha*, which means "to trust." To trust what is in one's own heart. To trust that the values you hold dear in your heart are ones with which you can confidently align yourself. Science, for example, is one of the things that I hold dear in my heart, along with honesty, humility, kindness, and the ability to apologize. Maybe faith is not that complicated. Maybe it is whatever allows us to keep taking steps forward when life gets hard—even when it is hard for years. Without faith, anybody hoping to heal from trauma and addiction is lost. To live with faith is a human birthright.

Faith is what allowed me to keep taking steps forward on my healing path when the fog was the thickest. And fortunately, the fog would begin to lift over time. Faith allowed me to work hard in the healing modalities that I was told would help me: therapy, new drug regimens, yoga, meditation, seeking the guidance of shamans and healers, and nontraditional approaches such as reiki and bhakti yoga, the yoga of devotion and love.

My story, at its core, is about faith. Not religious faith. A faith that is more human and essential. Faith in myself, a deep knowing in my heart and body that I was on a good path, an elemental trust that taking one more step forward would lead to where I needed to go without self-betrayal. A faith that, when the world pushed back and set me on my heels, maybe forcing me to backpedal, I could adjust my course a few degrees and then take another step forward. I had developed an understanding that if the universe knocked me on my ass yet again, I would be just fine. I would get back on my feet, dust myself off, and, leaning into the headwind, restart my journey with one more step forward. And another.

Luckily, I didn't know I'd need all the faith I had to meet the challenges of the next ten years. I still didn't know or fully understand that I was suffering from trauma. I was still under psychiatric treatment for bipolar disorder. But I knew on a deep level that I wasn't and never had been bipolar. I'd never been manic, and my depressions always appeared to be deeply situational. My anger didn't cycle; it grew almost exclusively out of my struggle with intimate relationships. And when the anger rose inside me, it felt ancient. I could tell it had little to do with the current situation. It came from the distant past when, as a child and teenager, I felt stuck in my family, at odds with its dominant narrative, and without options to save myself.

I passed road signs for Raton, the last town in New Mexico before you cross the border into Colorado. I'd driven the road countless times, usually with Di, to visit friends and family at various parks and ski areas in Colorado. Near the state line, the road climbs steeply on Raton Pass. In winter, the weather can get dicey fast. But this was summer, and so I would only have to worry about the storminess inside my own heart. As I left New Mexico behind and crossed into Colorado, my loaded-down truck began to heave and jerk. But I didn't flinch. I had faith. I pressed the accelerator all the way to the floor and shifted into a lower gear. I had faith, and I had desire. Not for material wealth, not for success, not for much that could be classified as "of this world." What I wanted was to feel healed and whole. To not live inside a fog of my mind. Maybe to travel again someday. Maybe to India again to connect with my younger self who'd been so awestruck by the murmuring *sadhus* in the Shiva temple. To see the monkeys climbing on the temple steeples. To watch the young boys fight the monkeys off and stand at the top of the steeples and leap as high and far as they could, forming an arc in the sky that no Olympic diver I'd seen could touch. To watch them splash into the Ganges below and disappear under water for two or three seconds. Sort of like I disappeared underwater in the River Jordan. And then appear again at the surface, not with anger or confusion, as I'd felt when I resurfaced. They resurfaced with big, beaming smiles and the most gleeful shouts to their friends up on the steeples, readying themselves for their leap of faith into the Ganges.

I decided that as soon as I got settled in my new apartment in Boulder, I would find all the trinkets and souvenirs from my world travels and place them on a shelf: a soapstone dragon carved by an Inuit man in Greenland; a black phallic candle given to me by a tarot reader in Manaus, Brazil, in the Amazon Basin; a bright red flaming heart made of tin bought at a shop in the Sierra Madre; a Ganesh statuette given to me by Di; and other items. I would look for a picture of Neem Karoli Baba on the internet and place it there, too. It would be an altar of my own making, full of objects that were meaningful to me.

Krishna Das groaned over the speakers. The cone-shaped, craggy, high peaks of the Sangre de Cristos soared to the northwest. My Ranger picked up speed. I made a wish. I wished Shiva would shatter me. Break me down to nothing, to pure soul essence, nothing more. So that I could build myself back up from the ground up. I wanted to disappear, but only for the sake of rebirth. I may not have believed in Jesus's resurrection, but I was going to believe in mine. I also had a second wish. I wished Gene Savoy could see me now; I was on a road going somewhere. Where, I wasn't exactly sure, except that I knew I'd be sleeping tonight in Boulder.

Six hours after I left Santa Fe, I passed Folsom Field, the University of Colorado's football stadium. I peered through the dark for the outline of the Flatirons, but the rain was too heavy on the windshield. The downpour was brutal, and some of the streets were flooded. I too was flooded with doubts and hopes and the overwhelm of moving—disoriented, but this time in a new way. The lights of the small apartment buildings lining Pearl Street flickered like votive candles at me through the rain.

I was driving through Boulder, but time became a loop, and now I was walking along the Ganges, gazing out at the flowery candlelit offerings. I was in between everything old and everything yet to come. I found my new apartment building and ferried my few belongs—a mattress, a couple of side tables, lamps, a coffee table, and a dresser—into my small apartment, and then I collapsed onto the mattress on the floor. I slept harder and more soundly than I had in a very long time. When I woke, I looked out toward the Flatirons, the craggy rock faces that symbolize Boulder's nature-loving aura, pulled on some pants and a T-shirt, and walked outside to survey the damage. Boulder was soggy but okay. So was I.

Walking the streets of my new town, I was still me, but I was fine with that. I walked and walked. A part of me kept looking for the familiar. Gone were the mud-colored, Southwestern-style buildings that had been my physical touchstones in Santa Fe. Gone were the restaurants touting chili-smothered enchiladas. Gone were the yellow chamisa bushes and twisting cholla cactuses, too. My gut clenched. For a moment, I felt scared. I felt a thousand miles from where I was supposed to be. I feared the return of the River. I fantasized about reuniting with Di and with Andrea—as if either of them would take me back now. I thought about the way I'd found moments of peace while walking the banks of the Santa Fe River. I admit, I also thought about loading up my truck and turning around and driving back. But I stayed. Maybe for the first time.

nineteen

ALTAR

THE SUN WAS SHINING IN BOULDER. THE EARLY SKY OVER THE foothills was salmon, and the clouds shone silver. The sunlight in Boulder was different than Santa Fe's. It was less brilliant and laser-like, but I fell hard for the glorious pink morning sky and the yellows and golds during sunset. I could see the streets of my new town were busy with runners, cyclists, and shoppers, but I had work to do to get settled. I'd moved just four hundred miles due north to another midsize city in the foothills of the Rockies, but on the drive up I had felt like I was crossing many time zones, maybe even continents. Only a few months earlier in Palestine, I was a journalist dipping his toe back into spiritual matters. But after going through my mother's death, another marriage and divorce, and traversing up and over Raton Pass, I'd crossed a threshold that couldn't be backtracked, into a territory without markings.

My to-do list was short but daunting. I was still taking a lot of medications that kept me foggy and unmotivated. I needed to establish care with a new psychiatrist who would, hopefully, see what I saw: that the bipolar diagnosis was a mistake. Dr. Jerry had handed me the prescription for lithium after a single fifty-minute session and subsequent psychiatrists had assumed that diagnosis was correct and continued treating me without casting any doubt. I'd later learn from both psychiatrists and therapists how commonly trauma was misdiagnosed as bipolar disorder in the 1990s and still is today.

I also needed to find a new therapist. How to pay for these essential services? We live in a time when psychiatrists and therapists—the good ones, anyway—accept cash only. And of course I had to eat and pay rent. I had no savings. I needed to find work. I couldn't risk freelancing again, pitching story ideas and waiting two or three months for a reply. My email to my brother David asking for a loan of a few thousand dollars to get my feet on the ground was ignored. When I texted him to see if he'd received it, he responded curtly: "I don't believe in your business plan." I had no choice but to trust. Trust what? Trust.

In my reading, I'd stumbled on Huston Smith's *The Stages of Faith*. The religious historian points out how the word "belief" has gotten twisted and is deeply misunderstood. Several hundred years ago, as Europe was experiencing the Enlightenment and science as we know it was being born, the word's meaning began to change. In thinkers like René Descartes and David Hume, Western culture fully embraced logic and reason. ("I think, therefore I am.") Science brought medical and technological advances that led to longer, healthier lives. But the changes came with a cost. Feelings were minimized and dismissed as less trustworthy than facts. Before the Enlightenment, "I believe" didn't demand an object, something to believe *in*. But now, to say "I believe" raises the question, What do you believe *in*? And the very possibility of believing in something as wild, mysterious, untamable, and *unnamable* as God went away—poof. Our language was washed clean of the ability to embrace the mystery of the universe, to not believe *in*, but to simply believe, without needing empirical proof. There's a reason why religious Jews spell God's name YHWH. Without vowels, the word is unsayable; God cannot be reduced to a word.

I will never get these boxes unpacked if I don't stop thinking and drinking coffee. Spiritual or not, I still had to unload the physical remnants of my old life. What did God's name have to do with clearing the fog, the brutal inner critic, the emotional windiness that kept me from finishing projects, kept me from staying in relationships, kept me locked in the past? I needed to focus on the present, with only furtive glances into the future. I removed four place settings of sky-blue Fiestaware from a box and set the plates in the cupboard. I took out my bright red Italian espresso maker and placed it on a burner on the stove. I unwrapped a full-spectrum lamp that I used in winter to try to chase the blues away. I unpacked my bathroom supplies: toothbrush, razor, beard trimmer.

And then I got around to my books. I'd given away most of my extensive collection before leaving Santa Fe. I kept only the books that were the dearest to me, the ones I thought of as my soul books: a signed copy of *Into Thin Air* with the inscription, "For Brad—With respect & admiration. Thanks (I guess) for your pivotal role in this book. If memory serves, it was you who first proposed sending me to Everest. In any case, I'm grateful for your assistance and sage advice you've provided over the years. Best, Jon Krakauer"; a signed copy of *Into the Wild* and the inscription, "To Brad & Di, With respect and admiration." Several *travel writing* anthologies, two of which containing my travel story about living in the woods with dilettante tramps outside Prague; *The History of Western Philosophy*; a biography of Carl Jung; *Man's Search for Meaning*, by Viktor Frankl; the Bhagavad Gita; Kerouac's *On the Road*; Peter Matthiessen's *The Snow Leopard*; Sharon Salzberg's *Faith*; Annie Dillard's *Pilgrim at Tinker Creek*; a book of essays by James Baldwin; Walt Whitman's *Leaves of Grass*, which I carried around in the glove box of my 1978 VW bus when I drove it from Kansas to Virginia and then up to Maine in the late 1980s.

After I arranged my books on the shelf, I made a quick tactical trip to Target to buy picture hangers and bathroom and kitchen supplies, all while dodging the people pushing carts full of jumbo twelve-packs of paper towels and bags of pre-battered chicken strips. Even from a dreary Target parking lot, Boulder was stunning. It felt more grounded than airy Santa Fe, as if the force of gravity were stronger here. My feet felt like they stuck to the earth when I walked. My body felt more solid, too. It might sound crazy, but I felt held by the massive granite mountains.

Boulder is a small city of a hundred thousand people that sits on flat land at the foot of the eastern slope of the Rocky Mountains. The

Flatirons, two brown-red blades of granite in the shape of irons, rise from the west edge of town. The next range over is Indian Peaks, and beyond that and a little to the north rise the high snow-capped peaks of Rocky Mountain National Park, including 14,259-foot Longs Peak, which I climbed as a skinny sixteen-year-old in 1982. To the east of the town is flat prairie land: mile after mile of green pastures, grazing cows, white farmhouses. It looks more like Kansas, where I grew up, than the Colorado of the movies.

A few years earlier, a Boulder homeowner dug up his backyard to install a hot tub and discovered thirteen-thousand-year-old stone tools that anthropologists identified as artifacts of the Clovis culture. Ancient wandering people came to Boulder to hunt ice camels. Later, the Arapahoe, Ute, and Cheyenne Indians occupied these lands, hunting buffalo, elk, and deer, until they were run off and killed off by white settlers who'd discovered gold in the mountains. By Boulder Creek, which runs through the heart of the town, is a sculpture of Chief Niwot, who cursed the area so that the natural beauty will cause people to want to stay, and "their staying will be the undoing of the beauty." The last big news from Boulder was the mysterious unsolved death of six-year-old JonBenét Ramsey, followed by a hundred-year flood and many destructive wildfires. Today, it's home to the University of Colorado, outdoor lovers, endurance athletes, and, more recently, tech industry start-ups. People come here for the beauty of the landscape, easily accessible hiking and biking trails, high-altitude training, and the abundance of spiritual organizations and teachers. On the surface, Boulder appears to be a paradise. But just like any place it has its problems: racism, poverty, and an ever-growing unhoused population.

Back at home, I was feeling antsy, so I took a break from moving in to walk along Pearl Street, Boulder's trendy pedestrian shopping avenue.

I stopped in a shop selling Indian religious figurines, tapestries, billowy pants, and saris. They were having a sale. I noticed a tarnished Shiva statuette, the type that adorns nearly every yoga studio in the United

States, in which Shiva is doing the *tandava*—a blissful, cosmic dance in which the universe is created, maintained, and resolved—on the back of a demon. I set the figurine on the counter and handed the clerk my debit card. She was an Indian woman who turned out to be the owner.

"Nataraja, very nice. You know the story?"

"No, I'm sorry. I don't. I just know he dances and keeps the universe going."

I was buying an object sacred to Hindus that I didn't understand; I felt suddenly ashamed of my naivete. The urge to buy this item far surpassed my desire to confront the critical issues of cultural appropriation that was symbolically, and literally, at play during this brief exchange. Still, I was focused on my sense that the world's religions and their symbols transcended borders. I was on a voyage inward, and Nataraja reminded me of that. My journey felt like a mission, an assignment both from someplace in me and from something far more intelligent and luminous than me. I was listening to a part of me that had been obscured, buried. It felt as wise and ancient as it felt new. Because it felt so essential and precious, I worried that I might lose touch with it. I felt I needed to pay close attention to my inner ear still and listen continually, lest I miss a single message. And the Shiva statue? One assignment on what I could tell was an extended, strange mission. What else was I going to be asked to do? Ignore the noise of the modern world and move toward things that spoke in words that our commercial culture had left behind. *Follow the feeling, Brad.* And this feeling, while positive in valence, contained a warning darkness too. It seemed to say, "Do not ignore me, or the price will be high." I had a strong sense that the cost of ignoring this feeling would resemble the scene at Paul's death. A body, cold and blue, lying on a cheap carpet in a dark hallway. The cost was death; if not a physical end, something just as final.

"This is going on my altar," I said. "I could use some Shiva."

She gave me a nod that felt like a signal of understanding.

I held the statue tightly on the walk home. Back in my apartment, now that I had toilet paper and sponges and all the necessary items you rebuy when you move, I could turn my attention to what I had seen all along, the most critical task of making my new home: the altar.

I'd never had an altar before. Di and I had sacred things scattered throughout the house: ornate Pueblo pots, tin-covered wood crosses made by local Spanish artists, smooth rocks from the beaches of northern Michigan, Di's home state. A gifted sculptor whose work was adored by celebrities like Oprah and Ellen DeGeneres, Andrea had holy things everywhere. Her Russian and French antiques felt holy to me. But, as I saw it, this was different. One of the pet peeves I have with the way people decorate homes is that the most crucial, soul-filled totems end up in closets or boxes because they don't fit the decor. This had always bothered me, so I was going to put the objects that meant the most to me on the altar. And the altar wasn't merely going to be something I fit into a convenient corner. This was the altar of my life. As such, these soul objects were going front and center. I placed a bookshelf sideways, tugged it to rest under the living room window, and wiped down the top.

According to Hindu legend, Shiva and Vishnu visited some monks in Tamil Nadu who had boasted about their ability to control the gods using mantras and magic. First the monks created snakes, but Shiva picked them up and wore them around his neck. Then they manifested a wild tiger, but Shiva killed it and wore its skin. Last, they displayed a demon, and Shiva stepped on its back and performed his dance of cosmic bliss. I looked at the statue. The words *fierce grace* came to me. One leg was held gracefully high; the other was planted fiercely on the demon's back. I placed Shiva at the center of my new altar. It felt right. I looked at it for a while. It anchored the other objects, and simultaneously I felt a solidness in my core.

There were so many commitments and good intentions I had not lived up to over my years so far. These things threatened the inner peace I was cultivating, threatened to convince me that this altar idea was just one more naive act. But I didn't care. I was resolute. I was listening to that inner voice. The altar would be the center of my universe, the focal point of my inner world. I put on some music and reached into a box.

I pulled out blue soapstone statues. One was a dragon, and the other, an Inuit hunter, purchased from an Inuit artist I met on my walks in Paamiut, Greenland. I set the statues on the altar. I reached into the box again and pulled out a fist-size brass statuette of Ganesh, a birthday gift from Di. Ganesh, the son of Shiva and Shakti, known as the remover of obstacles, is ubiquitous in US yoga studios. I dusted Ganesh off and set him on the altar. I reached in again, and my hand found a heart-shaped rock I picked up in the Italian Dolomites while visiting mountaineering superhero Reinhold Messner at his castle in Tyrol. I placed the totem on the altar. Next, I pulled out a wooden cross bought from a Spanish artist who lived near the famous "healing chapel" in Chimayó, New Mexico. I reached in again and grabbed a rosary I'd bought in Jericho. Next, a small, blue-flowered metal vase that held my mother's ashes. I cradled it in my hand. At some point, I wanted to scatter the ashes somewhere she loved, probably back in New Mexico. And then my hand found a long, wood incense holder. I rubbed my fingers over the engraved Shiva symbol. Shiva had been there all along. These objects, and others I'd find later in other boxes, were the remnants of my travels, souvenirs from real places inhabited by real humans, but that wasn't all. They represented the contents of my heart: my desire to find myself out there in the world. And although I hadn't found wholeness out there, these objects were dear to me. And as much as they existed in the external world on my altar, they were part of me, too. And they always would be.

Next, I brought out a gourd-sized clay pot I bought in the Sierra Madre Occidental. It was made by a Tarahumara potter who lived in the deep recesses of Los Cañones del Cobre, Copper Canyon, a system of six chasms deeper than the Grand Canyon, located in the southwestern part of the state of Chihuahua in northwestern Mexico. Was the map still inside? I reached into the pot. It was—a piece of white copy paper. One side had an elaborate pencil-drawn map. A friend of a friend who lived in Albuquerque had drawn the map to guide me from my house in Santa Fe to Urique, a tiny village at the bottom of one of the canyons. *But where's the heart?* I wondered. I reached into the pot again, and my hand found a palm-sized Sacred Heart made of tin, painted bright red with gold thorns and yellow-orange flames shooting out the top. Christians view this as the symbol of Jesus's infinite compassion for humanity, for all our flawed selves. I bought it from an artist in Creel, a logging town located at the tip of the canyons.

In my thirties, between 1997 and 2001, before I disappeared into my self-induced drug coma, while I was still conscious, I made several long road trips from my home in Santa Fe to those deep, intricate gorges. The first time I traveled with Craig, a college friend. Our mutual friend David was doing a postdoc in Urique, working as a physician. On the way down, we stopped in Albuquerque at the home of a friend of David's, who asked us to carry secondhand clothes and a water pump to some-body at the canyon's bottom. Since we'd never been to Copper Canyon before, he drew us a map—the map I just pulled out in my apartment in Boulder—while we sat at his table. He drew it utterly out of scale, meaning that the twelve-hour drive on the highway was short, and the dirt roads of the Sierra Madre took up more space. The distortion seemed not just appropriate for the circumstance but meaningful. The adventure took up more space than the routine.

I made the trip again a few years later, this time to Batopilas. I took the map with me again. The 780-mile drive took two days. The route be-gins on I-25 and shadows the Rio Grande until it reaches El Paso, Texas. There, I crossed the river into Ciudad Juárez. I slept in a cheap hotel with velvet curtains and red carpet pocked with cigarette burns. And then I headed straight southward on Chihuahua Highway 27, crossing the flat Chihuahua Desert with its mesquite and paloverde trees, cholla cactus, and agave and yucca plants, finally turning west on Mexico Highway 24 and then south on Mexico Highway 2 into the Sierra Madre Occiden-tal on a two-lane highway that changed from gravel to dirt through the pine forests. I passed rancheros, finally stopping at a house with a hand-painted sign that read "Comida." It seemed like a residence. I knocked. A woman in her thirties invited me in to eat an afternoon dinner. She was making burritos. Did I want one?

"Por supuesto," I said. "Si, tengo mucha hambre. Gracias!" *Of course. I'm very hungry. Thank you.* I was remembering my college Spanish.

I watched as she wielded a large knife and sliced a chunk of flesh off an animal's leg on the kitchen table. I assume it was a cow's, but it could have been a donkey's. She disappeared behind the counter and proceeded to chop the meat further. A few minutes later, she emerged from the kitchen, carrying a massive burrito smothered in green chili sauce. Whether cow or a donkey, it was the only food for miles, and it tasted delicious.

Eventually, the dirt roads led to Creel, the tourist entry point into canyon country. The area is home to the Tarahumara Indians, who run long distances while drinking a sacred beer and who became famous in the United States for running—and often winning—ultramarathons.

You can head in the direction of Urique or one canyon east to Batopilas. The roads into the canyon are steep switchbacks, with rock walls to one side and thousand-foot drops to the other, so narrow that each time you come to a car (or, God forbid, a bus) traveling in the opposite direction, both vehicles must jockey for position. The driver on the inside must figure out how to hug the wall without losing a side mirror. The driver on the outside must hug the other vehicle to avoid falling off the world's edge. Everybody driving these roads is generous and works hard to make it work; there's no option but to cooperate and do your best.

The drive to the bottom of the canyon takes more than four hours. But when you arrive, it's as if you've traveled thirty degrees farther south to the equator. When the temperature is 50 degrees in Creel, it can be near 100 at the nadir. The gorges aren't as wide as the Grand Canyon, but they cover four times more area and are deeper, as much as a mile in places. You wonder whether you'll ever stop descending. With each switchback, the temperature rises a degree or two, and the vegetation becomes increasingly tropical. It can feel like you're descending into the navel of the world. The two towns at the bottom are a bit different from each other. Batopilas is a tourist town with a Mediterranean-style white-domed hotel, a more modest B&B, and taco stands. Urique, a rustic old mining town, is far less touristy. These tiny villages are occupied by both mestizos and Tarahumara Indians.

Around the time I was traveling to Mexico, I read *The Teachings of Don Juan*, by Carlos Castaneda. Castaneda's books are mocked today as remnants of the 1960s, and he's criticized for fabrication and cultural appropriation, all of which are probably true. But those books, then and now, cast me into a trance. They speak about ways of seeing the world, ways of being in the world, that we modern humans, with our science- and logic-tainted minds, have lost touch with. Don Juan, a Yaqui Indian teacher, explains that humans once had the ability to shapeshift, or morph, into crows and coyotes and other animals, that there are many other realms besides this obvious physical one. He teaches how one can become a spiritual warrior by facing the four enemies: fear, clarity, power, and old age. I had my doubts about all this, but the teachings did confirm my returning sense—a feeling I'd had since I was a kid—that there was more to this universe than meets the eye. I didn't know if the specifics of what Castaneda said were true. That didn't matter to me. I knew he was right that there's more to the universe than our limited brains could make sense of. Perhaps all my travels, for work and leisure, were about trying to get more and more lasting tastes of connection with other humans, and maybe with the soul of all things. I think all of us have these feelings, but as we become adults steeped in our scientific, technological world, we learn to deny them. We pathologize them, like Dr. Jerry pathologized and tried to medicate my childhood mysticism. I had marked a passage in Castaneda's book, which I reread then, in Mexico, and years later, when I thought about my forays into Copper Canyon: "Anything is one of a million paths. Therefore, you must always keep in mind that a path is only a path. . . . Look at every path closely and deliberately. . . . Does this path have a heart? . . . If it does, the path is good; if it doesn't, it is of no use. Both paths lead nowhere, but one has a heart, the other doesn't. One makes for a joyful journey; as long as you follow it, you are one with it. The other will make you curse your life."

Did I know then—did I really know at a body level—that being an adventure writer was my path? Was working in journalism a path with heart? Had I made it so, or tried to? But was I living from my heart? I sometimes think that my collapse into the drugged-out fog of nearly a decade was the proof that I might have been living somebody else's life. But the 20/20 vision that comes with time is deceptive. Yes, I betrayed my heart in some important ways—and I also did the best I could.

The Copper Canyon region brought me alive in a way that few places in the United States have. The remoteness and the adventure were compelling, yes. But the land there, combined with its Tarahumara inhabitants, felt strikingly different to me from the Rocky Mountains of Colorado or even the canyon country of Utah. We Americans have mowed and cemented and built over damn near everything that once was sacred on our lands. Perhaps this is partly why we believe we must travel far distances to encounter the sacred, which in turns puts us at risk of exploiting other people and cultures. It's a huge mark of our privilege. And it also leads us to stop even trying to preserve our own sacred places.

When I went to Copper Canyon back in the late 1990s and early 2000s, I found that the Abyss didn't follow me to Mexico. Why? Because I went at my own pace. I wasn't representing a magazine or writing or thinking or worrying about a story, and I wasn't traveling for financial gain. I didn't have responsibilities. I never felt trapped. If I felt a little claustrophobic someplace, I moved on and quickly felt better. Nobody knew where I was. Nobody was expecting me. I traveled when and where I chose. I had agency. I had purpose and meaning, and I felt joy. All those things that were usually a part of my work travel made me feel trapped, like I was trapped on the log in the White River in Arkansas. But in Mexico, I followed my feeling. And when I followed my feeling, I felt at ease and deeply connected to the land, the people, and to myself. I felt at home despite being six hundred miles from my house.

I placed the pot with the map and the tin Sacred Heart on the altar. The Shiva statue was in the middle, near the back, and the other sacred objects now fanned out from this anchor point in a half circle. I strung beads over some of the icons and then, for the final touch, I added white Christmas lights and reached down to plug them in. Starry lights now encircled and illuminated each object. I lit a stick of nag champa incense I'd bought with the Shiva statue. As the smoke column rose, forming little eddies before dispersing into the four corners of my apartment, I sat on a pillow and stared at what I'd created: an altar. Not any altar. With these sacred objects obtained from the four corners of the world, I made a representation of my entire external universe, as well as an expression of my whole inner landscape. Both occupied the same physical space, all of it on one table, in a Target-decorated man cave at the foot of the Rockies. I had brought the world's soul, as I currently experienced it, into my apartment. I placed my palms together in a prayer position at my heart. I committed to myself: *Every morning, when I stumble out of bed, I will not pass Go before I sit at the altar. Wait, no, I will allow myself to make coffee. But otherwise, I won't pass Go. I will turn on the white Christmas lights, and I will . . . do what? Meditate? Pray? Practice yoga?*

I hadn't figured that part out yet. I would sit and pay reverence to whatever the hell was behind all of this. This world? The multiverse? Was there a universal soul? Did I have a soul? I was beginning to think I did—that we all do. And that the world does, too. But fuck if I knew.

The longer I sat in front of the altar, the more I wanted to cry. Then I was actually crying, and the longer I cried, the harder it was to stop. I was starting to feel the soulfulness, the meaning, the power that I felt in India, in Mexico, in Greenland—inside myself. I felt it around women I loved and women I slept with. I felt it listening to blues artists when I stumbled drunk into the Checkerboard Lounge on the South Side of Chicago in my twenties. It had always been outside me. And now it was here, right here, with me, in my apartment. So close it was almost like the power was inside me. Whatever it was I was feeling, the point was that I *was feeling*. There was no brain fog, no deflection, no escape.

I stood and walked through the apartment to see whether there was anything else left to do. It was mine, this place. There was no wedding photo on the wall, no golf trophies, no school photos of children. Instead, there were printed mandala tapestries, pictures of the New Mexico countryside, a photo of Bob Dylan wearing Ray-Bans. I admitted to myself it looked a little like a college kid's dorm room. And, of course, I had lost part of myself back in my teens, and I was going to have to work on growing up. But it was also a declaration. Part dorm room, part hippie vegan restaurant or opium lounge—I loved it. Whatever it was, it was mine.

Many years later, while I was still living in Boulder, my therapist, Susan, said something that deeply moved me. We'd arrived at a breakthrough: I stopped talking about my family and how I'd been wronged. I was focusing on stepping into a new life away from Colorado in a new city with a loving partner, a more thriving coaching business, and a more healed life. She paused the session and looked into my eyes the way she did when she wanted me to know that what she was saying was deeply true and that she wanted me to really understand with my body what she was saying.

"Brad, you have graduated. You graduated a while ago. But you need to know that you are no longer a child of your family. You are not the child of your specific parents any longer. You are a child of the world, a child of this universe, a child of God."

She paused and then spoke again: "Can you hear this? Can you feel it?"

I knew that she was correct. It had been true for a while, but I only knew it was true in my brain. It hadn't soaked into my body, into every cell. But at that moment, the feeling of belonging filled every organ, every cell, down to the mitochondria, into every corner of my body for the first time. Yes, I was a child of the world. A child of God. As such, I belonged! I may not belong in my family or in Kansas any longer, but I belonged to the universe because I was a flawed human who suffered. I pictured the crack in the Church of the Holy Sepulchre. I pictured the tomb where Jesus was laid to rest. I pictured the burning body beside the Ganges and the susurrating *sadhus*.

And back in 2013, as I returned to the altar I'd just built, after taking a break to wander and find some food, the sun set, casting shadows on my altar. As evening settled over Boulder, and the sky turned pink, I lit a candle and placed it on the altar. I felt a tinge of the belonging I would eventually experience. I had some difficult days ahead. I was bringing the journey of healing out of the landscape of foreign places and into myself. The work ahead wasn't out there but in here. The work was quite simply *to feel*. And for a few hours that day, I did feel: like I belonged. I felt faith. I was a child of Shiva, Ganesh, India, the Mexican Sierra Madre, Greenland, Indonesia, Russia, the Czech Republic, Israel, Palestine, Colombia, the Caribbean, the Brazilian Amazon Basin, Jamaica, Sweden, England, Kansas, New Mexico, and now Boulder, Colorado, and the front range of the Colorado Rockies.

If we are lucky, the incredible places we go will elicit deep, sacred feelings These places are worth celebrating because of the way they move us. But we also bring ourselves wherever we go. I brought Kansas, my family, and my childhood experiences to the places I visited. Sometimes, when I looked out over a vista, I could see only those things I carried. And I brought the places I visited—and all the karma contained in traveling there—home with me, too.

In the past I had brought my feelings of not belonging, and a message of not belonging, back home with me. But as I built my altar that day, I realized that maybe other things had stowed away in my luggage as well: the authenticity and community and histories of the world as I had experienced it. Yes, I *felt* wary of the potential for cultural appropriation, spiritual bypassing, and colonialism inherent in what was I creating. I'd read Edward Said, and I'd written about some of these issues in major magazines. But I also was convinced that this quiet act was decent and essential to my humanness.

The items on my altar weren't just objects; they were portals to devotion. Like a spiritual magpie, I arranged these talismans around me, sanctified them, and called this little apartment not only *home* but my place of prayer to belong to this wild, mystical world.

twenty

THE RIVER IS EVERYWHERE

I HAVE A THING FOR RIVERS. THERE'S THE HAUNTING WHITEWATER roar in my skull from the river in Arkansas, where I almost drowned. Roaring. Always. There was the house flooding when the creek swelled into a rising river, threatening to swallow us whole. In 1999, as a thirty-three-year-old adventure writer, I peered through the smoke of the burning ghat at the fiery corpse and into my soul, or something like it, on the banks of the Ganges. At age forty-six, I rebaptized myself in the aqua-colored Jordan River at the exact spot where tradition says Jesus was baptized. Throughout my nineteen years in New Mexico, my mind calmed while walking along the barely flowing Santa Fe and the fast, icy Chama. And there are more rivers. Rivers everywhere. The waterfalls I rappelled down and flooded red-rock slot canyons I swam through in southwest Utah. The still, flat kayaking waters of the Colorado River in the shadow of Hoover Dam. In college in the 1980s, my friends and I used to walk the metal catwalk under the highway at night and peer down at the swirling currents of the Kaw River in Lawrence, Kansas. I sometimes felt tempted to jump, not from a desire to die but to experience more . . . more than Kansas; more than the restrictive, conservative mores; more than the work-hard, study-hard life of a smiley, chronically depressed college student struggling to see the joy in absolutely anything. In 1997, I sat on a clump of grass watching the cerulean rivers that cut through Greenland's Icecap. In 2001, I stood on the deck of a houseboat motoring up the Amazon.

The air was like a wet blanket, and the river seemed infinitely wide, like it was everywhere. I watched the mermaid-like pink dolphins porpoising at dawn and the floating grocery stores and houses of prostitution at night. Rivers have traumatized me, and they have also healed me.

Back then, I wasn't conscious of my affection for rivers or what they might mean to me, what they did to me or might do. I moved toward them unwittingly, compulsively, as if I were a wand-wielding dowser, as if river-seeking code had been written into my brain's operating system. I was a diviner, drawn to water. But what did I want to divine? What did I long to know? Once, in Maine, I observed a diviner, an old man in a porkpie hat and a 1940s-style suit and tie, wander the piney woods holding a gnarled, Y-shaped stick. As he walked, the stick would wiggle and dip, apparently as he came closer to underground water. I wanted to talk to him. I had so many questions: Was this witchcraft or science? Was he a prophet or a fraud? But I held my tongue. I assumed he was the silent type, and he didn't say a word the one time I tried. Regardless, I was simultaneously mesmerized, doubt filled, and a 100 percent believer. Why not? Rivers appeared and then disappeared from my life. Or was it more willful than I remember? Was I always searching for my next river, like a landlocked fish desperate to breathe again?

In his 1914 paper "Remembering, Repeating and Working-Through," Sigmund Freud presented his idea of "repetition compulsion," noting how "the patient does not *remember* anything of what he has forgotten and repressed, he *acts* it out, without, of course, knowing that he is repeating it." Later, in "Beyond the Pleasure Principle," he expanded on compulsive repetition; he wrote that we have a "destiny neurosis," a built-in character trait that seeks expression *and* our destiny by neurotically repeating experiences. Freud's point contradicts the old saying that the "definition of insanity is to repeat the same behavior with the hope of a different outcome." He suggests instead that it is human to be drawn, over and over and over again, to what we consider our destiny or what will pull, or carry, or even drown us into our future.

Every morning, I woke before dawn. Always. Not because I wanted to but because sleeping rarely took hold for longer than four or five hours a night. Juiced up on coffee, I went outside and strolled the dark, empty streets. With each step, I imagined myself like Nainoa Thompson coaxing my own Easter Island, the island of my future, out of the black asphalt. As if pulled by gravity, I found my way to Boulder Creek, a small river full of icy snowmelt from the peaks to the west that ran hard through the center of town. This stream changed with the seasons: on snowy winter mornings it was cold, dark, and seemingly bottomless; in summer it ran swift and powerful and diamond-like. Whatever the season, the river became my anchor and a symbol of my emerging soul. It became my inspiration to clear the fog of my mind and step into my own power again. That was possible, right? Or had the drugs that blunted my emotions for nearly a decade done permanent damage? Was it my destiny to walk around forever in a stoned, zombielike state of mind?

The river told me otherwise. I walked the path beside it, sometimes striding, other times meandering. Occasionally, I stopped and sat cross-legged on a rock underneath an aspen tree, leaves clicking like cicadas in summer. I'd lose myself in watching the rushing, bubbling current. Over time, I became intimate with the water's orderly chaos. I learned to read its fluid shapes and differentiate its magic. The Vs where the moving liquid wrapped around submerged rocks and trout loitered; the swirling eddies where the water hurried to fill the empty space of a cutout in the river's bank, refuges for ducks; the clouds of swarming, just-hatched insects. On some mornings, a Zen-like tower of carefully stacked rocks would appear. On other days, I'd stand in the water up to my thighs and stack flat, wet rocks into Zen-like towers of my own. When I looked upstream, I saw the future. When I looked downstream, I saw my past. I stood, in the current, between them.

Could the river help me heal the Abyss and the PTSD flashbacks? Could I learn to move through the world with the power and grace of this river?

I began to draw energy from the river and to believe that I could find a new way to move, to flow, to be. I began to question the cruel doubt that arose in my mind as that repetitive, menacing question: *What is wrong with me? Why have I been depressed for so long? Why do I struggle to stay emotionally balanced?* Tracing the line from straight As and class president to living alone in a studio apartment after a second divorce and struggling to support myself brought up powerful feelings of shame. And sometimes, that shame made it impossible to move or to make a choice, which left me wondering and ruminating for hours, repetitively, compulsively questioning, walking, asking, wondering.

FORTUNATELY I ESTABLISHED CARE WITH A THERAPIST NAMED SARAH, whom I found very compassionate and caring and who seemed like a long-lost sister. She'd moved to Colorado from New Jersey decades earlier to be a ski bum and found herself studying Buddhism and psychology at Naropa. We were nearly the same age, and we both liked the Grateful Dead. I knew I had a lot to learn from her, and I began to unpack the story of my life, first once per week, then twice, in her neat, downtown office whose decor combined both elegant and hippie elements.

Eventually Sarah gave me the name of a psychiatrist: Dr. Benjamin. I made an appointment, but I was wary. I no longer saw psychiatrists or psychiatry as the answer to my problems. I didn't fear them so much as I feared me and my propensity to take what they told me as gospel. In the past, I'd trusted them and their diagnoses too much and my own judgment too little. At this point, I had doubts about the entire mental health industry—and with good reason. From my first session with a psychiatrist, I felt too quickly judged, pathologized, and medicated before the doctor even knew who I was. I felt as unseen by mental health professionals as I did by my own family. And the cost had been high: years in a drug-induced haze, life-threatening consequences of lithium toxicity, struggles with withdrawal, a therapist who slept through sessions. Much of this happened with my full participation, but doctors take an oath to "first do no harm." In my opinion, mine hadn't lived up to this oath. I had some very real fears to overcome. I tried to calm myself. I told myself that psychiatry was simply a tool I could use. Psychiatrists had a particular view of human beings, an idea that we were collections of diagnosable problems; their job was to figure out and name the problem and offer a solution in the form of medication. But I was starting to see myself very differently. I still needed their help because, let's face it, I still had a lot of problems. But now I refused to check my desire for self-preservation and autonomy at the door. I definitely wasn't open to hearing that the only solution to my real mental health struggles was medication. I knew in my body that going back onto large quantities of meds would be death. And that's not hyperbole.

A few weeks later, filled with fear, I knocked on Dr. Benjamin's door. I found the man who answered to be a kind, impeccable, dapper man with Ivy League bona fides, and he put me at ease. It took a few visits, but eventually I found myself relaxing my muscles and settling into the couch, but I didn't entirely drop my guard. I wouldn't for some time. From Philadelphia, Dr. Benjamin seemed just as knowledgeable about the science of mental illness as Dr. Winston in Santa Fe was, with one key difference: he was more skeptical about the *business* of mental illness. And he had a lot of empathy. I breathed deeply and relaxed further when at our third meeting he said this: "Let's get you off as many of these meds as possible, and then we'll see who you are." For now, a diagnosis was off the table. He said we needed to delve deeply into the effects of my having grown up with someone he had suspected was a narcissistic parent.

In all the years I'd been going to psychiatrists and therapists, this was the very first time the issue of narcissism had been raised, but after he explained the effects a narcissistic parent can have on children, I was curious. He recommended I read *Trapped in the Mirror: Adult Children of Narcissists and Their Struggle for Self* by Elan Golomb. Over the next few months, our discussions began to resonate. I now understand that many people who seek help in psychiatric offices are victims of narcissistic abuse.

They are the identified patient, or symptom bearers, of dysfunctional families. The problem with growing up in these families is that children weren't seen for who they are, and, on top of that, they are asked to be the emotional caretaker of the narcissist and the enabler. As Doctor Benjamin and Sarah assess it, all those days of pouring gin down the drain, worrying about our disintegrating family, and serving as my mother's emotional caretaker when she leaned on me for comfort and advice had warped my mind. These experiences rearranged my brain in its process of development. It wasn't just a state of mind problem. It was a brain problem. And healing the brain, rewiring the circuitry, takes time. And pills? Limited medications may be part of a comprehensive treatment plan, but they aren't the antidote. And the wrong pills at too-high doses can really get in the way of any healing at all.

I cried during these sessions. Both my therapist and my psychiatrist listened to me in a way that no one ever had, and I had certainly not felt as seen with any mental health professional. When I noticed the deep listening and care, I felt even more overwhelmed with emotion, a mixture of grief and relief at arrival: to safety, to myself.

Three months in and I was headed in a good direction, but nothing was solved. I struggled with cravings for the old meds and discomfort with the feelings coming through now that they weren't blocked. I felt like a teenager trying to live like a forty-eight year old. Fall turned to winter. By Thanksgiving, there was a foot of snow, and the temperatures plummeted to below zero. I had more and more productive sessions with Sarah and Dr. Benjamin. These appointments were the only social engagements on my calendar, and they helped with the loneliness. I had two people who cared about me and listened to me and truly supported me. But, man, good mental health support is expensive!

I found out about a writers' school for adults in Denver and sent in my resume. I was delighted to hear they wanted me to teach personal narrative writing. Within a few months, they offered me other classes. I hadn't taught memoir writing before, but I'd written and edited many first-person articles and essays. I embraced the challenge. Soon they made me the lead teacher for memoir in a two-year MFA-like program. I loved teaching and mentoring adult writers. It was fun and rewarding to turn the lessons I'd learned as a working writer into articulated craft lessons that helped others. I also liked being around people again. I'd found a community I could feel at home with. I received great student reviews. But, admittedly, I struggled with these new working relationships.

My own editing and writing coaching business was bringing in only a couple thousand a month. My psychiatrist and therapist bills were adding up to about $1,500 a month. The copays for a couple of the drugs I still took were $100 to $200 a month. And Boulder wasn't the most economical city for somebody mounting a life and career comeback. The one-time hippie town called itself the Free Republic of Boulder for its political and social liberalism, but Big Tech had arrived from the Bay Area, and there were a lot of people with a lot of serious money. The average home cost about $1 million, and I paid more than $1,000 a month for a 350-square-foot studio. But something there, in this place, felt right on a deep level that I didn't comprehend. I had things to learn there, and was I learning them.

I had a past, a troubled one, but I was learning that maybe I'd compounded the effects of that suffering. I medicated it. I traveled far and wide, hoping to escape it. I divorced when things got hard. I had built a life around running from pain, and in doing so I created a lot of suffering for others. I can argue that I grew up in a family that repressed feelings, hid secrets, and taught me to run from suffering. But I was also an adult, and I had to face these patterns within me and acknowledge my complicity in behaviors that were destructive to me and others. I had to let go, again and again, of the anger at my family. This proved to be one of the most difficult challenges I faced.

They did their best. Isn't that what we are meant to say about our problematic parents? I began to see the tragic nature of our family and the tragic nature of life. I had to assume that my father had forgotten his past, his tragedy. I suppose he needed to. I imagine his own psyche outright refused it. Yet I found for years I struggled with my own denial. I found it almost impossible to believe that a father, any father—my father—*willfully* denied his children a sense of reality that would have grounded us, a sense of reality that would have allowed me to understand my past and grow into a healthy adult. And yet this is what I came to believe, and it took many therapy sessions of dancing around this idea before I could fully accept it on a body level. It seemed morally reprehensible and outside the most fundamental duties of a father's job description. Or was he unconscious of his behavior? Whatever the truth, eventually I dug deep enough into my own psyche to punch through my denial about my father and family. I let go of my false hope that they would ever treat me with the love and respect that any member of a family deserved. In the process, I finally released a few fantasies about hope and how the world works too. The world doesn't hand out love or even acceptance. We must give these important things to ourselves.

Denial can be a hard pill to swallow. And my brother's role in the denial puzzled me too. I reached out to him more than once seeking corroboration, yet my texts, emails, and calls always went unanswered. I found this chilling. It sent me a profound message: I was alone in this process of healing. Worse, I still wanted their love. And that was the heaviest piece of all to let go of. I was a member of our family. Wasn't I deserving of some love? I guess I was, just as long as I didn't mention the past. But I couldn't fully heal if I kept playing my role in a dynamic that was destroying me. And so, I began my slow drift away. I imagined myself like David Bowie's Major Tom, with no alternate support system in sight. I could only hope for a better outcome than his.

Accepting responsibility for ourselves is the first step toward healing. But as much as the work is ours to do, we also need to trust others. We need doctors, therapists, and friends. And for somebody who'd lost the ability to trust others, this was a far more significant hurdle than it might seem. Dr. Benjamin and Sarah were helping me get over my anger at psychiatrists and therapists, but I knew I needed more good people in my life. My healing journey would have three prongs: trust in myself, trust in others, and trust in something greater than myself.

The river continued to be my anchor. The river flowed rain or shine.

In November, I took Dr. Benjamin's advice and adopted a dog. I found a gray pit bull mix at the shelter, and we fell in love instantly. A motley mutt, he had broken teeth from being kept on a chain, and his flanks contained five or six buckshot from a shotgun blast, but he was otherwise healthy and needed love, and I was ready and able to give it to him. I put him in a crate at home while I went out to buy him dog food. When I came home, he had dismantled the crate with his teeth and paws and was sitting on my bed. He seemed terrified of my potential negative response. "How could anybody be angry, Blue?" I said. "Don't worry. I get it." I tackled him lovingly, and we sat on the bed the rest of the evening and weekend, getting to know each other. I'd had dogs with Di and Andrea, but I loved this guy more than any dog I'd ever met. He was love. That's what he wanted more than food. He pressed his sausage-like body into mine when we slept. It would be a problem when I began to date, I thought. But I didn't care.

From then on, Blue and I walked the river together two or three times a day. In the evenings, we sat on my couch. He pressed close to me

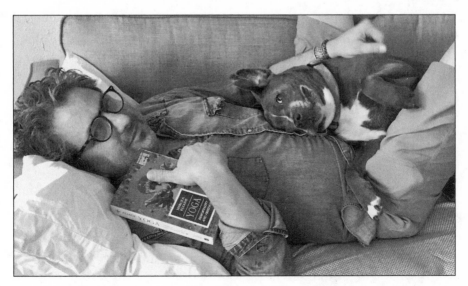

During our time together in Boulder, Colorado, Blue and I were inseparable.

as I read, mostly books about eastern spirituality and yoga philosophy: B. K. S. Iyengar's *Light on Yoga*, T. K. V. Desikachar's *The Heart of Yoga*, Sri Ramana Maharshi's *Who Am I?*, the Bhagavad Gita, the Dhammapada, and others.

The more I read, the more I saw that the Christian promise of a savior no longer seemed aligned with the world's reality, or at least not with mine. Eastern traditions encouraged humans to see and accept reality as it was: rife with suffering. The Buddha's central tenet was that suffering was baked into life. By accepting this—and the fact that we often create more suffering for ourselves when we attempt to run away from pain—we can find refuge in holding our expectations more loosely, gently. When we buy a beautiful new teacup, we can choose to see it as already having been accidentally knocked off the table and cracked. When we start a new relationship, we can see it as having already ended. The death of things is a part of the life of things. You cannot have one without the other.

The more I read and contemplated, the more valid the Buddha's thinking seemed to be. It was also at odds with American culture, with its unstated premise that we can buy and succeed and achieve our way out of suffering. But I wanted answers about my suffering. And I believed that the answers to these spiritual questions would also lead to healing. After a year in Boulder spent yoga-ing, meditating, and therapy-ing my ass off, I was ready to stop pacing beside the tributaries of spirituality. I was ready to ascend to the headwaters. Perhaps I was born to seek? Perhaps I would have been a wandering *sadhu* had I been born in India. Perhaps I was meant to live in a studio apartment at a subsistence level and seek It All like the Buddha himself.

One evening, I pulled my old, tattered high school copy of Hermann Hesse's *Siddhartha* off my bookshelf. I hadn't read it since I was eighteen years old, and now I was stunned by the story's effect on me.

A young Indian man grows up privileged and sheltered. He sees suffering outside the walls of his palace and realizes that there is more to the world than living a protected, privileged life. Leaving that life behind, he becomes a seeker, *sramana* in Sanskrit, wandering for years with his friend Govind. The *sramana* movement began around 600 BCE, around the same time that India began to experience urbanization. Then, Indian spirituality centered on the Vedas, texts controlled by the Brahman caste. Spiritually inclined men began to doubt the authority of the Brahmans, and the Vedas, too. These seeking *sramanas* left the cities and wandered the countryside, living in forests and caves. They experimented with spiritual practices they hoped would lead to more profound spiritual truth and understanding. Some of their methods were outrageous by modern standards: standing up twenty-four hours a day, hanging heavy weights from their testicles. Others became the practices of pranayama (breathing) and postural yoga.

When I came to the end of Part 1, when Siddhartha meets the Buddha teaching in a grove and realizes his teachings weren't what he was looking for, I wept. This is what Siddhartha says to the Awakened One:

> The teachings of the enlightened Buddha contain much, it teaches many to live righteously, to avoid evil. But there is one thing which these so clear, these so venerable teachings do not contain: they do not contain the mystery of what the exalted one has experienced for himself, he alone among hundreds of thousands. This is what I have thought and realized when I have heard the teachings. This is why I am continuing my travels—not to seek other, better teachings, for I know there are none, but to depart from all teachings and all teachers and to reach my goal by myself or to die. But often, I'll think of this day, oh exalted one, and of this hour, when my eyes beheld a holy man.

SIDDHARTHA MEETS THE BUDDHA, AND WHAT DOES HE DO? HE WALKS AWAY FROM HIM. Why? He knows he must continue his journey. He must find the spiritual truth for himself. He must trust his own body, his own senses. The Buddha wasn't his path. Siddhartha's life was his path.

"'I shall no longer be instructed by the Yoga Veda or the Aharva Veda, or the ascetics, or any other doctrine whatsoever. I shall learn from myself, be a pupil of myself; I shall get to know myself, the mystery of Siddhartha.' He looked around as if he were seeing the world for the first time." There were many habits, ideas, and even people I needed to walk away from. It seemed next to impossible to peer through the fog of my mind and figure out what should stay and what should go. Some days, I fantasized about becoming a *sadhu*. I'd wander from temple to temple, living on handouts and eating from trash bins. Could I get by on alms? It was pure fantasy, obviously. On days when I was able to think more clearly, I saw how impractical, how ridiculous, how impossible—and how terrifyingly lonely—such a life would be. An American *sadhu*? I'd probably be laughed off the subcontinent. And yet, I resonated with Siddhartha's need to walk away from the Buddha—from everything.

While the book explores Eastern spirituality, it is a decidedly Western book, too. Siddhartha is an individual who decides he must go on his journey. It's about Western individuality as much as it's about Eastern wisdom. I had read it once before, during the last semester of my senior year in high school in Prairie Village, Kansas, when I was a depressed Izod shirt–wearing naïf who, like my friends, believed a great college was the answer to everything. Maybe it soaked into my unconscious because I became a seeker, and one who couldn't commit to any path. Wandering, seeking spiritual answers, but never able to land in a place of belonging and commitment. Nothing quite fit.

In Boulder, weeks turned to months and then years. I quit teaching at the writing school. Through fear-based, impulsive, reactive behavior, I'd turned the administration and the staff into my dysfunctional family of origin and myself into the scapegoat. I naively told myself it didn't matter because the school paid poorly, and so I wasn't keeping up with my bills. I focused on building my editing and coaching business. I also took my car to the shop for a tune-up and signed up to drive for Uber and Lyft. I drove late at night and early in the morning. I drove tech CEOs to Denver International Airport. I drove drunk college students home from the bars. I didn't mind. I turned it into another spiritual practice like yoga and meditation. As I drove, I listened to Krishna Das. I listened to Buddhist podcasts. I longed to see India again. I was working as many hours as I could, given that I was still fighting the fog and low energy. My monthly haul was barely $3,000. I told myself to remain patient. *Do the work. It's bound to get better soon.*

Rain or shine, no matter how exhausted I was, I woke daily at 4:45 a.m., and I walked the creek with Blue. Boulder Creek got fat and thin as rains and seasons came and went. Some days, Blue and I kept on walking. We walked right out of town and up into Boulder Canyon, split in two by a four-lane highway that often closed by rockfall. We crossed Canyon Boulevard and found the trail to Boulder Falls, where I sat on a flat rock. I watched and felt the cold spray of the falls for a few minutes. I caught glimpses of the way I hungered for intense experiences. I felt like I couldn't get enough of the roar and the cold spray against my hot skin. I longed for more: more experiences, more wholeness, to feel more connected to life.

We enter the world as sponges, don't we? Babies, which we all were once, are very focused on the external world, specifically on their parents. When a child is treated with love and care and kindness, they learn to trust that the world will provide for them, that the world values and wants them. Eventually, hopefully, this experience becomes internalized, and a child learns to carry this sense of being loved inside themselves, wherever they go. I think this looks like trust, maybe even like faith. Children who grow up without positive parenting become adults who are externally focused. We seek validation, safety, and faith *out there* instead of reaching inward to access it. We suffer. Because these learned ways of being in the world stop serving us in adulthood. We become addicts, or seekers, or, in my case, addictive seekers.

I needed to confront this particular addiction that I believe led to my overmedication. I pledged to go to Al-Anon meetings. I made other pledges. Hibernate in my apartment less. Get more exercise and spend more time in nature. Build community with other humans. The spray from the waterfall was starting to chill me, so I made my way home, down Boulder Canyon. I cooked a healthy vegetarian meal. I called a friend from high school. I challenged myself to do different healthy things that weren't second nature to the housebound man I'd become.

From the autumn of 2013 to the winter of 2017, I lacked a formal diagnosis, but I did everything in my power to experience healing. Therapy, psychiatry, daily yoga and meditation, walking in nature, dog love, building friendships and community. They began to have their effect on me.

I'd let go of things, too: my tendency to isolate, my habit of fixating on the past. After a yoga class, Taylor, a warm, inclusive yoga teacher who was also a psychotherapist, drew a cartoon Brad. And around it, she wrote "yoga," "therapy," "Taylor," "Ram Dass," and "spirituality." She handed it to me to look at. Her point was obvious: I was the center of my world. It was new to me, as somebody who'd been codependent all my life. Aren't we supposed to put others first?

It was the first time I realized the paradox of spirituality and psychological healing. Psychology and spirituality were connected. They were related. But they weren't the same. Their relationship was paradoxical. If I listened to Ram Dass and focused on serving others now, I would bypass my own need to build strength and resilience. I had grown up with a weak sense of self, so weak that I sometimes felt like I didn't exist late at night when the Abyss opened up. And although I still didn't have a prescriptive mental health diagnosis, I was okay with that for now. I gave myself my own new diagnosis: human. I kept my eye on the task at hand: reclaiming my body and mind—my soul.

What if emotional and mental suffering had simply been my karma? Could I cling less tightly to the details, to blaming my difficult family and my former doctors, and instead accept that mental illness was simply my path? Maybe I could see my family challenges in a fresh and perhaps more liberating way: it was what was given to me. In my reading I learned the word *dharma*, which roughly translates to "purpose" or "path." Our dharma is related to our karma. If mental suffering was my karma, my dharma was healing and maybe eventually being of service—perhaps helping others heal? Maybe. But first, I had to heal myself.

I sometimes lost myself in my studies of yoga and Eastern wisdom. I became obsessed. It's what I do. I fell down the rabbit hole, and for a time, I sought to achieve higher states of consciousness. But I knew better, too. My experiments with ecstatic states of *samadhi* and *nirvana* were short lived. I returned to doing my mantra and loving-kindness meditation for twenty minutes twice a day. I also experimented with other types of meditations. One meditation recommended by trauma specialists is "box breathing," which I later incorporated into my daily routine. In box breathing you inhale slowly, counting to four, focusing your attention on the sensation of the air entering your nasal passages and down into your lungs. At the top of your inhale, you hold your breath for four counts. Then you exhale for four counts. At the bottom of your breath, you pause your breathing and count to four. You can try this for four minutes at first. If it feels okay, you can extend the time.

In the winter of 2017, Dr. Benjamin told me he was leaving town. I wept when he hugged me and said goodbye. He handed me a piece of paper with the name and phone number of Dr. Marc, another Boulder psychiatrist he trusted. I called and made an appointment.

I was feeling stronger. More so every day. I was hiking regularly in the foothills near town, and I felt ready for a bigger adventure. I planned a trip to Longs Peak, in Rocky Mountain National Park. I'd climbed the 14,259-foot mountain with my brother in 1982 when I was sixteen, a highlight of my youth. I didn't expect to get to the summit this time. I merely wanted to climb above tree line, maybe stand at the feature called the Keyhole and peer through it to the jagged peaks on the other side. Maybe the point was to feel as alive as I felt at age sixteen. I might have been depressed at that time, but I also felt a full range of emotions. I wasn't a zombie. Like Frankenstein's monster, who knew he came from human parts but wasn't fully human, I craved feeling fully alive. What could be wrong with that?

I left my apartment before dawn one late August morning. The aspen leaves in the national park were turning gold, with smatterings of orange and flaming red. The air smelled of vanilla mixed with cinnamon and coconut, the scent of the sap of ponderosa pines being warmed by the sun. I breathed in deeply. The cool fall air filled my lungs, and I imagined breathing in all the way to my toes. I'd just read an article online about the healing properties of spending time in nature. I already knew this, of course, but I felt affirmed by what I read. At *Outside*, nature's healing properties were the subtext of most of our articles. Humans are animals; we are part of nature despite having surrounded ourselves with urban jungles made of concrete and steel. Getting outside more was a part of leaning into healing modalities, all of which were necessary if I wanted to continue reducing my medication intake. With all the beautiful options available, hiking was an obvious ritual to fold into my routine. This plan seemed to make good sense.

I looked up at the canopy of the aspen grove as I walked, the leaves of these strong trees linked together by deep and elaborate root systems, turning from green to gold, a truly magical time in the Rockies. I took another deep breath and imagined the fresh air cleaning out the synapses in my brain and the tiny capillaries in every corner of my body. I imagined the air mopping up toxins in the very mitochondria of every cell. I listened to the pleasant chattering of blue jays and ground squirrels and the ornery caws of ravens. By now, the angle of the trail had steepened, and I was breathing harder and sweating. But honestly, it felt good to challenge my body.

I kept walking. The trail crossed a small, clear stream and ascended at a steep pitch through a pine forest. The golden-white light became muted and green-gray. I noticed that I was walking faster, despite the incline. Suddenly I felt like I was running from something or someone. But from what or whom? And, equally important and confusing, to where? I put my hand on my chest to feel each beat of my heart, which pounded against my sternum like a heavy metal drummer. I wanted to stop, I could have stopped, but instead I kept walking. The forest was getting thicker, and the gentle golden light that had lit the path through the aspen grove was now largely blocked by the dark green pine canopy. I was not even a mile away from my car, but I felt very far from civilization.

Paranoid thoughts began to infiltrate my mind, which was peaceful just moments before. What would happen if I got injured and couldn't walk back out? *Oh, be quiet,* I told myself. *This is a popular trail. Dozens if not hundreds of people hike it every day. You will be fine.*

That was all true, but I wasn't okay. Fear began to take hold. I felt anxious, and then scared, and then I felt the Abyss. I laughed. *You are one mile from your car, Brad. Keep hiking. It's good for you.* I remembered how I'd calmly faced heavily armed Israeli soldiers at checkpoints. I spent ten years adventuring all over the world: traveling a thousand miles up the Amazon River, rappelling down waterfalls and swimming through narrow flooded canyons in Utah, paddling a long stretch of the Colorado River. I'd camped on a ridge overlooking the Greenland Icecap and lived with dilettante hobos in the woods of the Czech Republic. And more. And yet, I didn't understand how those far-flung excursions had traumatized me. And so I was frustrated to be so unsettled by this local, well-traversed hiking trail.

I stopped in my tracks. I felt a creeping inner darkness that was matched by the disappearance of the direct sunlight out in the open canyon. I craved the bright gold-white light again. I felt the outer darkness seeping into my body and mind. I grew fearful that the shadows would usher in sadness, maybe full-blown depression, and the brutal inner critic that accompanied my dark periods. I was done with that inner critic, but dismissing it filled me with absolute terror. Who would I be if I failed to listen to it? Would I even exist? What if I got in its face and said, *Go fuck yourself?* Would that work? Or would the voice only grow more aggressive and bullying? I couldn't take another step.

I'm confident the shift in light was more subtle than it felt. But even the sounds of the birds, the wind, and the river seemed nefarious, as if the natural world were full of danger and out to get me. I felt like

I was entering the mythical black forest where people encounter evil spirits and the creatures that inhabit nightmares. And then the river in Arkansas came roaring back into my head. The beach in Greenland, too. And the panic attack in the plane over the Atlantic en route to the Czech Republic. I wasn't sure I'd be able to walk the mile back to my car. Paranoia set in. I thought about being attacked by mountain lions and psychopathic murderers. What if I had a heart attack? Hyperventilating, I turned around and walked toward the car. Then I started to jog.

I ran for thirty seconds or so but quickly became breathless and couldn't sustain that pace. I began walking like a racewalker, all herky-jerky. I felt too embarrassed to break into an outright run. There wasn't any real danger out here, right? Right? When I spotted the visitor center and then my car through the trees, I slowed down and breathed a sigh of relief, but another neurotic fear quickly replaced this: *Jesus, I hope my car starts.* Once inside, I locked the doors. I took a swig from my water bottle, ran fingers through my hair, and looked in the rearview mirror. *Who am I?* Wasn't I a world-traveling adventure writer who wrote for the very best magazines in the country? And yet I can't even go on a short walk in the woods on a Sunday morning. Am I a fake? Have I lived a false life? I remembered the many times that my father and brother had made cutting remarks and called me what I feared most: a fraud. I remembered posing in front of the inflatable Dos Equis bottle as they laughed and snapped pictures and called me the Most Interesting Man in the World. Were they right? Was I a coward who'd wrapped himself in a false image as a brave adventure writer? Had my entire career been the story of a coward who so needed to see himself as brave that he tortured himself until he collapsed into a ball on the couch?

At this point in my life, I hadn't yet received the diagnosis of trauma from two psychiatrists and three licensed psychotherapists. I had no idea why my mind and body reacted so severely when I entered nature or why I couldn't escape those looping thoughts. But now I understand it better. I experienced—endured—immobilizing, terrorizing emotional flashbacks on that hike and indeed on every adventure-writing assignment

I'd gone on. These episodes grew worse over time. Each time I ventured into unknown territory and felt these intense feelings of fear and outright terror, I added another layer of trauma over the previous. By now, I had so many layers of trauma that I couldn't even take a hike in the woods without suffering a near-total emotional breakdown. I was reexperiencing It All. I felt only shame that morning, coupled with the strong sense that my writing career had been a lie. In fact, I believed that my father and brother were right and I was a fraud.

I drove back to my apartment. I got Blue, and we walked down to the river. I sat cross-legged on the rock, but I felt like lying down and rolling up into a ball. *Will you fucking relax!* I screamed inside my mind. *Why can't you just take a hike like a normal person?*

I had released a lot. I saw my mental suffering as my karma, but suddenly hopelessness was back. That night I drove Uber until two in the morning in a blur. I was too numb to go home and too tired to call anybody. I found myself alone at a gas station, buying packaged crackers and cheese. The app on my phone showed a bank balance of $194.00. I was doing everything right. I was showing up for myself. I was showing up in the world. But the fucking universe was not showing up for me. I was self-pitying and furious. I was getting better, but now I was regressing instantaneously into a two-year-old. Even Dr. Benjamin was perplexed in the end. In our last session, he said, "You definitely don't have bipolar, Brad. But I don't know what is going on here. I'm thinking more along the lines of trauma. I think you and Dr. Marc will figure it out. For now, I'm calling it 'adjustment disorder.'"

"Adjustment disorder? What does that mean?" I asked

"Nothing really. It's sort of a catch-all. It means that a person has a strong reaction to major change. I have to write something in the box. Don't think about it, Brad. I believe you'll get to the bottom of this with Dr. Marc."

A lifetime of suffering and three years of work with Dr. Benjamin, and this was the end result? "I don't know"? "Adjustment disorder"? I tried to follow my breath and settle. It worked—sort of.

I eventually went back home, and Blue and I collapsed onto the bed. *When will this purgatory end? Will I ever pull out of this?* Suddenly I felt as alone as I did on the glacier in Greenland. I turned on some chanting music by Krishna Das. I breathed. I cried.

Three weeks later, I sat in Dr. Marc's office and retold the story of my life. I went there once a month for the following year. A year defined by editing, driving Uber, and yoga. And walking the river. I was doing everything I could to heal. I wondered when it would be enough. I wondered what healing would be like and feel like, and how I'd be able to tell when it arrived.

At the end of *Siddhartha*, we find our hero aged and sitting by the river. "The river is everywhere," Hesse writes. Those words still choke me up. The river is everywhere. That river in Arkansas is never far from my mind. Its roar is a permanent fixture in my psyche. The way the river pushed my skinny body into the log and, at the same time, pulled at my limbs downstream, trying to free me. That push-pull dynamic was everywhere. When I was alone. When I was in a relationship. When I was in community. My pathology threatening to drown me, my faith trying to save me. The river was indeed everywhere, all the time, every moment, every day.

When Boulder Creek was low and the weather cold, I walked into Dr. Marc's office one January day, almost a year after we began our work together. I sat down. He took out his pen and notebook. As I always did in doctor's offices, I inhaled nervously. I put up my guard in case he planned to tell me something that didn't feel true. And then I exhaled. Within the hour, my life would be changed forever.

twenty-one

REAL FAITH

DRIVING FOR RIDESHARE SERVICES IS PERHAPS NOT AN IDEAL way to make a living. After paying for gas and wear and tear, I made about ten dollars an hour during the three years I drove for Uber and Lyft. And the hours are not ideal either, especially for an early riser; the best time to drive in a college town is late at night, when the students want to escape their dorms for the bars. So that's when I drove. Just as I was in the mood to curl up on the couch with a cup of tea, my dog Blue, and a book about the history of yoga, and then stumble a few feet across my studio to my bed to crash for the night, I instead warmed up my little Kia Soul and switched my Uber and Lyft apps to "available." I was a fifty-year-old man driving carloads of sorority and fraternity youth, and, more than once, I found myself at the car wash at 2 a.m. vacuuming vomit off the back floor. If I was too tired, I occasionally left the dirty work for later in the morning. But Boulder is cold at night, and cleaning up frozen vomit is next to impossible.

That's how I began Christmas Eve 2017. And after I cleaned up the vomit, I took out a brush and cleaned up the dog hair. I loved Blue so fiercely that I was happy to deal with his fur.

Through the icy back window, I could see the rock faces of the Flatirons. In the snow, these slabs looked like a frosted cake at a forty-five-degree slant. I listened carefully for the *ping* indicating a passenger had summoned me to pick them up for a ride—hopefully to the airport.

Come on, airport run! I thought. Airport runs paid about seventy dollars for the hour and a half of driving—compared to trying to link several short rides at five or six dollars a pop. *Damn, Blue's hair is fine,* I thought. I knew I probably shouldn't let him ride in the car while I was driving for ride services, but I liked taking him with me everywhere. *Fuck, who cares if my passengers get a little blue-gray fur on their slacks.*

Ping. The sweet sound of money. I looked at my phone. Jennifer wants a ride. Let's see. Where does she want to go? To Walgreens on 28th. Where does she live? Two blocks from Walgreens. *Well, hell,* I thought. I accepted the ride and prepared to smile when I saw her. I hit play on Spotify. My car filled with the sound of a harmonium, a small, portable pump organ used in sacred Indian music. Then a baritone voice joined, singing words in Sanskrit, the ancient, sacred language of Hinduism, Jainism, and early Buddhism. "Narayan, Narayan. Om Namo Bhagavate Vasudeva," which I knew was a holy mantra that could be translated, "I bow to Vishnu, the Sustainer, the god in all beings." I sang along because it's a catchy tune. But I'd also learned that many Indians believed that reciting this and other mukti mantras brought liberation to the singer. I felt in deep need of liberation. Pretty much every Western method I'd tried had not helped much. So, why not chant? Krishna Das was about all I listened to these days. His chanting had become the soundtrack of my life.

I took off past the bungalows of Walnut Street and over to Pearl and its trendy boutiques and cafes, then to Broadway, which runs parallel with the mountains. I took a left on Pine, pulled over to the curb, and pressed the button on the app to tell Jennifer I'd arrived. She indicated that she was running a few minutes late, so I put the car in park and waited, amping up my singing, wondering what my next passenger might be like. When Jennifer appeared, I was surprised to see that she was an attractive woman in her forties wearing yoga garb. As she opened the door, I turned down the stereo. And off we went to Walgreens! I waited in the parking lot with the car running for ten minutes while she shopped, and then I drove her back home. I closed out the ride and checked to see how much I made: $3.20.

Well, it's a start. I'm building character, I told myself, half-jokingly. *And this healing journey requires* tapas. *Tapas*: Sanskrit for "heat, fire, discipline."

In Patanjali's *Yoga Sutra*, a spare document written between 200 BCE and 500 CE that is essentially a how-to for ascetics about being in a state of *yoga*, or union, the author, a mystery even today, shares the eight limbs of yoga—basically the eight aspects of a yoga practice. *Tapas* is part of the second limb of yoga, Niyamas, a list of observances or internal guidelines: *saucha* (cleanliness), *santosha* (contentment), *tapas* (discipline), *swadyaya* (self-study), and *Ishvara pranidhana* (surrender to God). I was working on cleanliness and contentment. They weren't natural to me but seemed attainable. Self-study did come naturally to me—maybe too much at times. The surrender to God part seemed like the final step; I wasn't there yet. But *tapas* I thought of as the theme of my life right now: I needed the discipline to sit still in the fire and the intensity of the journey.

Since moving to Boulder four years earlier, I had applied myself earnestly to healing and personal growth: weekly psychotherapy; daily yoga, meditation, and journaling; studying addiction recovery and going to Al-Anon and Co-Dependents Anonymous meetings; and reading about Eastern spiritual philosophy. I had talked weekly with a habit coach / spiritual counselor named Joshua.

I *was* healing and growing.

I had completed a two-hundred-hour yoga instructor training and was a budding teacher of postural yoga. I taught yoga classes and journaling for self-growth for free in the park along Boulder Creek.

And the healing and growth journey was continuing. I spent two or three hours each morning in silent spiritual practice in my apartment. I spent evenings driving Uber, a job that was like a spiritual practice because of its requirements of humility, patience, and, yes, *tapas*. My writing coaching business was picking up, too, though it often took a back seat to my self-growth and spiritual development work.

And although I wasn't seeing results that anybody on the outside would call tangible, I didn't care. I wasn't tired of the hard work. I knew patience was part of the journey. I had faith that my work would eventually pay off. And in the unlikelihood that it didn't? I had faith in myself.

I wasn't spending all my time alone. After years of self-isolation, I had a handful of new friends, people I respected and who respected me. Chris, a nonfiction writer from New York City; Paul, a novelist from Pennsylvania; Tamra, a therapist from Chicago via San Francisco; Gillian, an aspiring memoirist who'd taken classes from me; and her husband, Mike, a corporate marketing executive; Stephen, a photographer, and his wife, Leigh; Dave, a magazine art director with whom I'd worked at *Outside*. Gillian and Mike opened their home to me for Sunday night family dinners. And there was Amalia, a passionate social worker and single mother from Vermont. She and I tried dating on and off, and while the romantic chemistry was there, and I felt I loved her, I couldn't commit for reasons I didn't understand. Amalia saved my ass more than once late at night with her kindness and care when the Abyss showed up.

I tried my hand at dating. I wanted to find Ms. Right, but I couldn't seem to meet a woman with whom I felt the ease that I'd enjoyed with Di and Andrea. The new relationships always faltered after a few months and sometimes after a few sleepovers. I seemed not to understand the secret of midlife dating. I didn't quite see how my situation contributed to my dating woes—how residing in a cave-like studio apartment, driving Uber, and talking exclusively about spiritual matters could be liabilities in a town where most women my age, I assumed, would be looking for wealthy tech executives. But I didn't care. I also discovered that, if all I wanted was sex, being a poor, fucked-up yoga teacher wasn't necessarily a liability. I had no problem in that area. The problem was, sex wasn't all I wanted. Looking for Ms. Right kept me in a cycle of short-term, occasionally *very* short-term, connections. In one therapy session, Sarah strongly suggested that I had become a sex and relationship addict. I didn't believe her at first. In one morning session, I boasted giddily that a woman I met at the cafe I occasionally visited had asked me to come over on this morning, immediately after my therapy appointment.

"For God's sake, will you have some dignity, Brad?" Sarah said.

"You know, women objectify men as much as men objectify women."

"Your point?" And then I got it. "Ah, you mean, you think women are sleeping with me just to have sex? But they don't really want to *be* with me?"

"I would slow it down, Brad. Yes, they would. I think you are a sex addict, and you are meeting a lot of sex addicts." I now understand she was right. A hundred percent. As soon as one fling ended, I felt the Abyss creep in, and I immediately returned to the dating apps and swiped till I found somebody new. I didn't feel okay in myself if I wasn't spending time with a woman.

And so, I tried to turn my focus away from sex and relationships to business. I signed up for a few one-on-one sessions with a business consultant. He encouraged me to slow down on the spiritual seeking and pay more attention to my business of editing and writing coaching. "I was like you ten years ago, Brad," he said. "All I did was meditate. I finally realized that if I wanted a better life, I needed to spend that time working on my making a living. I think you should do the same. Your yoga teaching? I'd stop it if I were you."

I didn't think he was wrong—but I didn't know he was right. I knew that I would have to make practical changes eventually, but I loved teaching yoga. I saw it as a spiritual practice that took concentration and gave back to people. And I was aware of my addictive tendencies and the possibility that spiritual seeking was an addiction for me. I now see spiritual seeking as an addiction if you seek enlightenment, certainty, and an end point. But if the seeking is seeking more of you, I don't think it is pathological. Because it was during these years that I became the person I am now. I'd always considered myself outside the mainstream. I objected to US materialism, but I had participated fully in it—partly out of necessity, partly out of pride, habit, and training. The whole nine yards, including a mortgage, a car payment, and nice things. By going so deep into spiritual seeking, I created a nonmaterialistic life for myself, whether I wanted it or not. The humble, simple place I finally found myself in—one of my own creation and borne of conscious choices—felt good. It felt solid and real to me. With less on my plate, I could understand and relate to my surroundings in a new way. With a smaller, quieter life, I could finally start to see the causes of my own thoughts and actions, and their effects on the arc and quality of my days and nights.

And yet, in some ways, my small, quiet life wasn't a choice. I couldn't have worked a regular job with my foggy state of mind. And the little secret that I didn't tell anyone: I spent at least three hours a day napping. The man who'd burst out of the gate of his career and traveled the world on assignment, working long days and sleeping short nights, had difficulty working at a computer for two solid hours without collapsing into bed afterward. There were health-related reasons for this, including that I'd slept only four or five hours per night for as long as I remembered, but the essence was that my entire being was exhausted. I was trying not to dissociate, and that work alone was exhausting. Maintaining a sense of full presence required staying in my body and harnessing my mind. I was still working to taper my meds, so my body was in a constant state of adjustment. Yoga and meditation were slowly but surely helping to bring my body and mind back online, to access the inner strength and energy I hadn't had since . . . ever? But it was slow going.

By the fall of 2017, I began to waver. I wondered—sometimes obsessively—where I was headed. I cringed to think that I would spend the rest of my life learning about healing and spirituality and then approach death realizing I'd spent my life on self-help, and to what end? It seemed beside the point. I began to see that maybe there wasn't an end point to this healing journey.

Can I let up a little with self-development and start to live again?

The Buddha and the yogis seemed to offer me interminable, unattainable lists: the Four Noble Truths, the Eightfold Path, the Three Characteristics of Existence, the Four Boundless States, the Five Hindrances, the Ten Perfections. On and on. There was always another list, another practice. It seemed endless. Was there a quantum leap I could take? I didn't so much ask myself this question overtly; it was bubbling below the surface.

Then again, I certainly wasn't looking for the easy way out. I began to doubt that my approach was going to let me know when I'd arrived. Would I know when I was healed? What would a healed Brad look, feel, and act like? When would I start to love me?

One day, I sat on the picnic table outside my apartment building reading the *Yoga Sutra* and writing notes. I came to Sutra 1.23–24. Patanjali tells us that if you wish to still the mind without wasting too much time in the process, then take a shortcut: surrender yourself entirely to God.

Wait a minute, I thought. *I wasn't expecting this.* I had been feeling overwhelmed by yoga and self-analysis. My approach was starting to remind me of how I used to overresearch and overanalyze every article I was writing until I thought in circles and couldn't find the story. Maybe simple was better. Like Occam's razor: the simplest solution is usually the best. I closed the book in frustration. Here I was, earnestly trying to learn all these dos and don'ts, and now it was telling me I could simply "worship God" and love. And how was that supposed to heal me, I wondered?

I was so ignorant.

Today I understand that love is the way we heal. Love is the most healing medicine on the planet. Ram Dass talked to me about love daily through my car stereo.

My guru didn't teach anything. And that was frustrating. I asked him, how do I raise my kundalini [spiritual energy]? How do I become enlightened? He said this: Love everybody, serve people, and remember God.

He said that romantic love is not real love. Love happens inside us. Love is twenty-four hours a day. Love radiates from within like the sun.

I loved all this talk of love. And though I'd worked so hard at healing and relearning how to be in healthy relationships, I suppose I wasn't ready to absorb this message fully.

Instead of loving myself, instead of easing up on myself, I doubled down on yoga. It had helped so far—it really had. But I was attached to it as the solution instead of as a tool that was serving me along the way. I clung to it like a log in the river. Some days I went to two heated yoga classes a day. I began seeking only women interested in yoga on the dating apps, as if that was a workable strategy. Looking back, I needed something to shift. I needed to slow down.

And then, one night, as I sat on my couch, scrolling the streaming services for something to watch on my laptop, I saw a documentary about Krishna Das pop up. I'd spent countless hours listening to his music, but I knew surprisingly little about him. And I'd never heard him speak beyond that 2001 concert in Santa Fe. I hit Play.

The documentary began with his three years in India with Neem Karoli Baba, who was also Ram Dass's guru. Then it followed him back to the United States after Neem Karoli Baba sent him home. Krishna Das fell apart. He began abusing drugs, specifically freebase cocaine. He knew he was on his way to an early death. His life turned around in the 1990s after a mentor he met at the ashram confronted him during a visit to the States and ordered him to stop using drugs. He did. He understood he needed to return to his spiritual roots. He began chanting at a yoga studio in New York in the early 1990s, and, over the course of years, as yoga took off in the United States, so did his music. He was nominated for a Grammy in 2013, and he sells out small theaters to this day.

The documentary moved me profoundly in ways that I didn't understand. The forested mountains of the Himalayan foothills, the white and red steeples of the ashram, still photographs of a young Krishna Das. He sits alone by a river. He walks, dressed like a *sadhu*, across a narrow bridge over the Ganges on his own. He admires his avuncular guru in a group of smiling hippies. He meditates next to statues of the gods wrapped in flowery garlands. It took me straight back to India, before my psychological and medication-infused collapse. And as soon as it was over, I played it again. In the days that followed, I played it sometimes two or three times a day. I ate breakfast while watching it. I fell asleep with it playing on my phone. The movie became my next addiction. Something about Krishna Das and his story hit me in the heart. The way he sought answers to life's big questions, the way he overthought his life. His inner strength. His humility and irreverence, too. His swear words. Underneath his talk about unconditional love, I could sense a vicious inner critic within him that he obviously grappled with and maybe halfway tamed. Our falls and comebacks looked entirely different, of course, but I sincerely felt a shared experience with depression, addiction, and spiritual seeking. And we shared a love of India and Ram Dass.

Krishna Das's effect on me during the following months reminded me of my teenage obsession with Jesus. If Jesus was the dad I didn't have, then Krishna Das was the older brother or uncle I would have loved to have: a compassionate man who thought and felt deeply about the types of things I cared for. He had tried to find meaning and answers to life's biggest questions; instead, he found love. Looking back on that early obsession with Krishna Das, I think he represented myself to me. The me I wanted to be. The me who was coming back from addiction, depression, and disillusionment through wisdom, yoga, and chanting; who was getting closer to feeling healed; who was looking to stop being so obsessed with healing and instead to feel more healed—who was looking to live again. I loved how he spoke about how our thinking can be the problem because overthinking can be addictive. Chanting, like other spiritual practices, organizes our minds and bodies. It rewires our brain and reconnects mind to body. It calms the churning of thoughts and quiets our minds, which leaves room to feel God. Which leaves room to feel love, from the inside out, just as Krishna Das said his guru allowed him to feel.

One day on a whim, I googled Krishna Das's concert schedule and learned that he was playing nowhere near me in the next year. But he was playing soon in Encinitas, California. I hadn't been outside Colorado since I moved there. I added up the expenses: $200 for a flight, $180 for two nights at the Rodeway Inn on Highway 101, $40 for the concert and a half-day workshop. I was there.

Perhaps I was off on another messiah-chasing adventure, but this one felt different from the rest. On faith, I bought the plane and concert tickets. Out of love for myself, I booked the motel.

The two-day kirtan workshop took place in a large concert hall filled with several thousand people at the Center for Spiritual Living, an ecumenical spiritual community. I arrived two hours early for the first night: a kirtan concert. Like a giddy fanboy, I sat on the floor near the front of the hall with the other Krishna Das junkies. I sang along loudly and clapped my hands. My heart felt like it would burst. After the concert, I crashed hard in my room at the Rodeway Inn. The next afternoon, I sat on the floor again and listened to Krishna Das tell stories about his years in India with Maharaj-ji and describe his realizations on his journey of healing and transformation in the fifty years since.

It would be dramatic to say that that workshop was "transformational" for me. I don't believe we can change overnight—real change takes new habits, new mindsets, and time. And I was working on those things. As I listened, I was reminded of all the books I'd read, the YouTube videos I'd watched of Thich Nhat Hanh, Pema Chodron, Jack Kornfield, Sharon Salzberg, and others. I remembered going to a talk by Ram Dass twenty years earlier and writing down a few quotes in my notebook, which I still had on my bookshelf. With time, I added other Ram Dass quotes to the notebook until it was full, and I began a second notebook. On this night, this quote stuck out to me: "What is it you want in this lifetime? What is it you want? You try to optimize pleasure and minimize pain. You try to get high and avoid the low. You say everything in my life, the highs and lows, is grist for the mill of going home. And it's even farther out than that, because at that point, your suffering becomes functional for your awakening. You're suffering literally becomes grace. That's a heavy one."

Yes, that certainly is a heavy one. A difficult teaching, to be sure. I realized how absent this kind of wisdom was in our culture. How long

I'd sought to connect with men who spoke from the heart like this. I rarely heard high-profile men, women, or anybody speak with deep wisdom. All I cared about was living from this depth of truth. That's what I wanted. I wanted to live from the depth of me, from truth.

Krishna Das peppered his teachings with self-deprecating humor. During the Q and A, he offered tough love to people who seemed to need it. One man complained that he felt tortured because he was trying to "bring more of the god Krishna into his life." Krishna Das's blunt response: Stop worrying about Krishna and go home and fix your life. Set goals for what you want, and work hard to achieve them. In other words, don't let spirituality keep you from living a healthy, prosperous life now.

I realize today that I wasn't drawn to him because he taught. It was the opposite. His workshop was an unteaching, an unraveling, a coming apart. He didn't ask the crowd to believe anything he said. He asked us to stop using our ruminating, thinking brains. The bottom line of all his teachings: Stop thinking so much. Thinking too much is a prison. "You can't think your way out of a prison made of thoughts."

Can I let go of my thoughts? I doubted it. *Can I turn down the volume?* I thought maybe I could. Krishna Das proposed a way to do this: "Open your heart."

Around this time, I began reading about the heart, both its scientific and spiritual aspects. I came across the work of the late University of Hawai'i neuropsychologist Paul Pearsall. He wrote extensively that our cultural fixation on the brain has robbed us of our ability to see the heart as a place of intelligence and wisdom, a flip he likens to believing that the sun orbits the earth. When I read this, I called my friend Dr. Ted Burns, a neurologist at the University of Virginia, and he confirmed that the heart does contain millions of neurons similar to the brain's and thus it could be thought of as a center of intelligence. These discoveries supported my gut feeling that Krishna Das wasn't speaking New Age bullshit. Jesus and the Buddha taught this too.

As Krishna Das wrapped up his workshop, I realized something important. My Holy Land journey had tried to teach me this lesson about the heart, too, but I wasn't ready to hear it then. The heart is how we heal. The heart is where our humanity lies.

Too bad I'd developed my entire personality around my intelligence. I had protected myself from my family by developing my thinking brain. The only way I knew how to shine was to try to outthink my brother and father. But I also used my intelligence competitively around others. I was good at providing the right bit of information, something I'd read, to cap off a conversation and prove my dominance. I'd weaponized the thinking brain and turned it into a bully. It hadn't helped me make friends. It hadn't served me in romantic relationships. I wanted out of the prison of my thoughts and into the freedom of my heart. Krishna Das said that many internal and interpersonal conflicts resolve themselves if we cease seeing them as intellectual problems and move our attention from the brain to the heart. Of course, the brain is important, too. But the great yogis, Jesus, and the Buddha knew something that modern-day people have largely forgotten: the heart and the brain can be trained to work together.

"Some problems dissolve with practice," Krishna Das said, referring to meditation or chanting. "So, go home and practice. Don't read about it. Don't talk about it to your friends. Do it. Or not. It's your choice."

Krishna Das closed the kirtan with a prayer spoken while playing a quiet, humble-sounding chord on his harmonium:

> If we know anything about a path at all, if we know that there might be a way to live in this world in a good way, with an open heart and without fear, it's only because of the great beings that have gone before us, out of their love, out of their kindness, they left some footprints for us to follow. So, in the same way that they wish for us, we wish that all beings everywhere, all of us, be safe, happy, that all of us have good health and enough to eat, and maybe we all live in peace, and that ease of heart . . . that ease of heart with whatever comes to us in life. Shanti means peace, peace beyond all understanding. When we know who we are, when we live in the love that

is within us, then we know that we are peace. May we all be that. *Om, shanti, shanti, shanti.*

On the way out of the event, I walked up to Krishna Das, shook his hand, and thanked him. I fought back the tears. I knew that he'd heard words like mine a thousand times, yet I had to say them. "You have no idea the effect you've had on my life. No idea."

"Thank you, but I don't know what to say. I just sing to Maharaj-ji," was his response.

After the workshop, I walked the beach, allowing the surf to wash over my feet. I thought about what Krishna Das said. On the plane home, I tried to temper my enthusiasm about it all with the full knowledge that I was chasing again—chasing gurus, chasing messiahs, chasing chanters. I was acutely aware of my habit of going down rabbit holes, of losing myself in the teachings and charisma of other spiritual gurus, especially men. At home, I rededicated myself to my practices. I devoted the next phase of my healing journey to moving deeper into my heart. Was I even a journalist anymore? Who was I becoming? This journey was entering a new phase that I could not have predicted, and I wanted the heart with . . . all my heart.

As I settled back into my apartment, I hugged Blue often. We walked the creek. I needed to be gentle, to guide myself into my heart gently. I followed Krishna Das's advice. I chanted more. I put my hand on my chest and felt my heart. I was aware that my healing journey was getting a little esoteric or that it might seem that way to others, but we live in a society that doesn't honor this way of being. I felt I had no choice. I remembered those lines from Carlos Castaneda that I reread during my trip to Mexico: "Does your path have a heart? If it does, then it is good. If it doesn't, then it is of no use."

As grounded as I was trying to be, being in Krishna Das's presence planted the thought in my mind that I needed to return to India. Soon, it was all I thought about. I had first seen Ram Dass speak in 1999. I heard Krishna Das chant in 2001. Neither event had a major impact on me. In

2010, I began listening to Krishna Das's music. Around that same time, Andrea's friend Janis shared *Be Here Now* with me. I still wasn't hooked. And now, watching the documentary in 2017, I was blown away. Why now? Why not then?

What I wanted more than anything was to travel to India, to the valley where Neem Karoli Baba's ashram is, even though the guru had been dead for forty years. My desire somewhat baffled me. India was next. I knew it. Yet I also knew it was a little off the wall. Remember, I was a journalist, or at least a former one. I was, and am, a natural skeptic as much as a spiritual seeker. I didn't tell many of my friends about my plans to go to the dead guru's ashram to try to retrieve my soul. I felt clear and confident—even joyful about my life and what was next for me.

And then, in December, I sent a letter home at Christmas. I'm not sure why I did this, why I let my guard down. Today, I ask myself, *What did you expect, Brad?* In the letter, I shared my journey of spirituality. I told my family about how meaningful my travels in Israel and Palestine had been, and I expressed the anger I held toward my former psychiatrist, my better situation now, and my dream of going to India.

That Christmas, I was alone in Boulder. I had been dating a woman for a while, but it ended. I found being alone on Christmas meaningful. I was learning to love myself again. I woke up and walked Blue and drove for Uber. It was slow. Boulderites were up in the mountains skiing. I went to a friend's house for Christmas dinner. And then I headed out to drive again. I drove most of that holiday week, though passengers were few and far between, and I made less than $200. On New Year's Eve, I attended a party at a friend's early, then drove until 2 a.m. On the forty-minute drive home from downtown Denver, I cranked Krishna Das louder than ever. I sang along with him. "Hare Krishna," "Baba Hanuman," and "Om Namah Shivaya." Could I feel my heart now, I wondered? If I kept at this heart work, would I feel it more next year?

A few days after New Year's, I called my cousin Paul, one of the few family members I have a warm connection with. He said he was at the family holiday events back in Kansas. Then he said something that made my heart drop all the way down into my belly.

"They read your letter out loud at Christmas dinner," he said. "Your brother sent it to a psychiatrist."

I didn't understand. I thanked Paul and hung up as the anger started rising in my body.

My father and brother had read my private letter to the people gathered at a holiday event—to my extended family and to *strangers*.

When I calmed down, I saw this episode as more information. I thought I knew exactly why my brother did it. He needed constant affirmation of my mental illness to reinforce the narrative that I was the fucked-up one. Why? Because it let him avoid looking at his own life and limitations. I began to see my family differently. I'd spent my life practically worshipping them, even when we fought. I'd seen them as super-healthy and me as the sick one. I finally saw through the trance I'd fallen into during my lonely childhood. They might be as fucked up as me, maybe more so. It wasn't my emotions that I had to overcome; it was them. Perhaps they were emotionally stunted people who protected their egos and made themselves right by making others wrong. *You can't become emotional, Brad. If you do, there must be something wrong with you.* Emotions = bad was the arithmetic I grew up with, the arithmetic I believed in until it nearly destroyed me. My father's favorite line was, "I don't do drama." Yet he brought more drama into our home than any of us. Perhaps we were all equally messed up in our different ways?

Moreover, my father had made a living representing men in divorce proceedings. One of his clients, a high-profile Kansas City–area businessman, had a series of ex-wives, all of whom were "crazy" and wanted his money. I imagined my father's conversations with them: "All my ex-wives are crazy, and they're trying to steal my money." "Okay, let's ensure these crazies don't bother you." Had he ever considered his client's role in the dynamic? I remembered the few times he offered me dating advice. "There are a lot of crazy women out there."

I never heard my father question the sanity of a man who got married and divorced a half-dozen times. Or say that guy needs to do some work on himself. I never knew my father to go to therapy or express that he needed to shore up parts of his character. My father was a card-carrying member of the patriarchy—powerful men using their power to put down people who didn't show loyalty to their authority.

I coped with this episode with more yoga and more meditation. I talked on the phone with Joshua, a spiritual advisor in the Bay Area whom I'd begun working with. I called old friends from high school with whom I had reconnected. I was creating more community. In Boulder, I found a sweet community of people at Raj, a small yoga studio. My teacher Taylor Moffitt's following consisted of middle-aged men and women who'd been through a lot in life. She emphasized living authentically, embracing our messiness, and emotional sharing more than the traditional eight limbs of yoga. I fell into this group, and suddenly I had twenty or so fellow seekers. I was finding home.

And yet life was hard. One blustery January afternoon when the sky was steel gray, I took Blue on an afternoon walk on Pearl Street. As we passed a cafe, a large pit bull–mastiff mix pulled free from his owner and attacked Blue so viciously I thought he would be killed. The other dog took Blue's entire skull in his mouth and bit down hard, intent on crushing it. My heart sunk. Adrenaline coursed through my veins. I kicked the attacking dog in the ribs as hard as I could. I grabbed its tail and pulled like in a tug of war contest, but I couldn't coax its release. I was certain Blue was going to die. Desperate, I lowered my shoulder, and put all my strength into kicking the attacking dog under its muzzle. Stunned, the strange dog released Blue's skull. Before it could turn against Blue and me, the other dog's owner appeared and grabbed the leash and tugged his animal away. I picked Blue up into my arms and ran toward my apartment. I threw him into my car and drove him to the vet. Thankfully, the vet's examination revealed only deep cuts and bruises. My fear that his skull had been crushed or cracked were unfounded. Blue spent the next week hiding in my clothes closet, but he was okay.

And then, one night, I cuddled Blue on the couch when I felt sick. I guess I'd never had a full-blown case of the flu before, because it astounded me how ill I got. Two weeks later, I thought I was better, and I resumed driving for money. But then I had the terrifying sensation of feeling my lungs fill up. I couldn't breathe. I was weak. I went to urgent care and was diagnosed with pneumonia. I spent the following weeks stumbling down my stairs to pick up food that my friend Gillian dropped by for me, struggling to breathe. Thank God for Joshua. He mentored me in grounded spirituality. He emphasized that we must trust in ourselves and maybe the divine, too, but we don't even need to understand the word "divine."

Laid out on the couch, unable to walk, drive, do yoga, or speak, I had to face some facts: I had become a consumer of information about healing and spiritual enlightenment. I had read more books about spiritual matters than any person I knew. I lived and breathed self-help and spiritual growth. I was filled with the opinions and methods of gurus, but I had no clue what I actually thought or, more important, felt, or how to put those teachings into action. I spent my life looking outside myself, seeking first success and then peace of mind, never really venturing to discover the truth that was already within me. Pneumonia slowed me down. As I lay on the couch next to Blue, struggling to breathe, I saw my life more clearly. These new realizations brought tears—and humility. I cried because I saw myself, maybe for the first time. I was just a baby on the spiritual path. I wondered whether, during my lifetime of seeking "out there," I'd stuffed down parts of me that I was afraid to deal with: fears, resentments, self-doubt, envy. All in my quest to feel better. I had confused personal growth with trying to become somebody I wasn't and could never be. It was becoming apparent that the next, and maybe the final, step in self-growth is self-acceptance. We must let go of the fantasy that we can meditate or yoga our way to being somebody else. We will never wake up in the morning as that different person we've been trying so hard to become.

twenty-two

FEAR AND TRAUMA

W HEN I FINALLY STARTED TO FEEL WELL ENOUGH, I dragged myself to Dr. Marc's office, even though I could still barely breathe. I'd been seeing him for about a year, and generally it was going well. He had only seen me in my new, less-medicated state. He was gruff in appearance and personality, in contrast to Dr. Benjamin's tidy warmth. Dr. Marc looked to be in his sixties. He still wrote prescription refills on paper, which he sent to patients through the US mail. He had strict rules about contacting him, which he enforced ruthlessly. He was decidedly old school.

But he was also decidedly modern in his caring and personal approach with me. First with Dr. Benjamin's guidance and now with Dr. Marc's, I had weaned myself off most of the drugs that Dr. Winston back in Santa Fe had prescribed. Now, I took a more straightforward, perhaps common regimen of medications: a medium dose of an antidepressant; a med to treat the fog of trauma, which can look like ADHD; and a microdose of Abilify, one of the antipsychotics that Dr. Winston had put me on that I couldn't seem to eliminate from my regimen, as hard as I tried, without going into severe withdrawal symptoms, including the sensations that bugs were crawling inside my legs when I tried to sleep.

Each time I visited Dr. Marc, he asked the same questions: How are you doing in general? How is your mood? How is your business? How are your relationships?

I would take a deep breath and tell the story of the past month. To be honest, in retrospect, I wasn't doing that great in some ways, even years into my self-care regimen. I was still unbearably lonely at times, I was still doing a lot of online dating, and it wasn't going very well. I was seeking a life partner but behaving like a sex addict. For one thing, I told him, I seemed to choose women who had many of the same issues that I did. I'd fall in love too fast, after one or two dates. We'd sleep together immediately. The sex would be hot and compulsive. And then, after a few weeks of bliss, the arguing would start. If we worked through to the other side, we would have makeup sex for a few days, and then the arguing would begin again. One of us would walk out with a door slam, and then one of us would panic, and we'd reunite. It was Toxic with a capital *T*.

Dr. Marc cautioned me to slow down, to be careful in choosing who to sleep with, and recommended an initial thirty-day period of celibacy before jumping into bed. I nodded, but I knew I probably wouldn't be heeding this particular aspect of his advice.

In addition to relationship issues, I was having health issues, I told him. Yes, there was the pneumonia, but after that passed, my blood pressure went through the roof. I was experiencing a lot of body pain that didn't seem to have a cause. I slept only about four hours a night. Most disturbing, I had pain deep inside my back, along my spine, that reminded me of the pain I'd felt for two weeks after the canoeing accident. MRIs showed nothing, but the pain persisted, and I couldn't sit straight. I felt a little silly telling him all this, but honesty had been working so far, so I admitted to him that I was worried that all these issues portended the onset of a significant disease—MS, ALS, or worse.

But my report wasn't *all* chaos and carnage. I told him about my consistent daily yoga and meditation practice. These activities had done what no drug had been able to: they calmed my nervous system so that I felt more at home in my own body. I felt a more solid sense of myself, even if these modest gains weren't showing up in my relationships yet.

Having covered the usual topics of my mood, my work, and my relationships, Dr. Marc set his notebook down and looked at me. "It's been a year of working together, and we haven't talked about diagnosis, Brad," he said. "I haven't wanted to go there with you because of your history with psychiatrists and diagnoses. But I think it's time. I think it will be helpful."

My balls constricted into my abdomen like they had the morning of the canoeing accident. I braced myself. I wanted to hear what he had to say—and I also didn't. I breathed in deeply, sharply, and then again more calmly, and exhaled. I put my hand on my heart and reminded myself how far I'd come and that his was just an opinion.

"Brad. You have post-traumatic stress disorder. PTSD. Your case is complicated. You have trauma from your childhood. You have trauma from your career as a travel writer. You have trauma from how doctors and psychiatrists have treated you."

I couldn't breathe now. Every muscle in my body was tensed, as if I had been shocked.

"I'm so sorry you've been through all this," he went on, slowly. "You never had bipolar disorder. You don't have a personality disorder. Brad, I'm sorry for all you've been through. I apologize on behalf of my profession."

I sat there motionless and stunned. At first, his words landed like a shotgun blast to the heart. Too much too fast. And then, as the word "PTSD" swirled around and around until my brain caught up, I breathed out and felt a moment of relief. But relief was short lived. A tsunami of emotion surged through my entire body. The feeling burst out of my gut, shot up my chest, neck, and face, and burst out my eyes as tears. I was overcome by every emotion—and all at once. I was worried I might cry harder than would be acceptable, even to someone who had seen me cry many times before. I felt ashamed.

"Brad, you can cry without covering your face. It's okay."

My hands dropped to my thighs, and I wept, and wept, and wept.

I had been seeing Dr. Marc for more than a year; he'd seen all my divergent sides, all my emotions: grief, anger, sadness, dissociation. I'd even lost my temper at him a few times. He knew as much about me as anybody on the planet. He knew more about me than Di, my friends, my colleagues. He knew far more about me than my family of origin—which was a pretty low bar, I guess.

"Brad, I have some advice for you. I hope you will take it. I want you to take a note card and write these words on it: I will always take care of Brad first. I will not betray myself to please anybody, especially my father and family."

I nodded my head in agreement. "I promise I'll do this."

"Okay, good." He handed me a tissue. "Our time is almost up."

I began to gather the notebook and pen I carried into each session.

"Brad, one more thing. I'm so proud of you and the hard work you're doing. I really care about you." A couple of years later, when I moved away, he'd even say, "I love you."

I began to weep again. Today, merely thinking about this moment, his words, still makes me cry.

I left his office, drove back to my apartment and stretched out on the couch. It was a pathetic little place. I was fifty-two years old, and I lived, worked, slept, and practiced yoga in the amount of space most Americans allot for an entertainment room. But it was all I needed. I lay there for a few hours, holding Blue. I was exhausted. I also felt something I had little experience with: contentedness.

And I was hopeful. Healing from trauma was a path, a path that would take me somewhere, as Gene Savoy might say. It was as if, for half a century, I'd been trying to navigate Mars using a map of Earth. Dr. Marc just handed me a map of Mars. It was still going to be rough going, but at least there would be a foundation of truth underpinning everything.

Later that evening, I drove Uber and Lyft for a few hours. On the way back from an airport run, I spotted the nubby summit of Longs Peak a few degrees to the right of the sunset. I recalled climbing it in 1982, when I was sixteen, scrambling hand over hand to reach the top with David, my brother. That night, I felt deep satisfaction with what he and I had accomplished together. I drank my first beer, and I connected both the accomplishment and the beer with becoming a man—something I cast doubt on today. But regardless, I felt strong and alive and deeply connected to that mountain. I felt a wholesomeness that perhaps only comes from spending time in nature. A few years later, when I was twenty-one, I climbed similarly difficult peaks in Maine and New Hampshire, and I led six or seven fifteen-year-old boys up them. I taught them how to camp and cook in the wild. I taught them how to respect nature and themselves and each other. Late at night, we talked about what it means to live a good life. We shared our dreams, fears, and hopes for the future. The memories added to my sense of inner strength and the narrative that I was a decent human. A human who loved the outdoors then and could love it again. I could get over the flashbacks when I hiked. I knew I could.

I hit a pothole, and I was jolted back to the present moment. I realized where I really was—not on Longs Peak, but in my Kia Soul. Those memories were just memories. Everything except what was happening in this moment, inside this Kia Soul, on this highway outside Boulder, Colorado, was nowhere to be found anywhere outside my own thinking. All I had, all that was real, was my breath and this moment. The first line of Patanjali's *Yoga Sutra* was clear about it: "Atha yoga anushasanum," Now begins yoga! Yoga begins now! Let go, Brad. Let go! Live in this moment. Live again! And get yourself back to India and recover your damn soul, for god's sake.

As the lights of Boulder got closer and brighter, I could feel the other side. The other side of what? I had no idea, but I felt a grounded hope, grounded in a way I'd not felt before. In Dr. Marc I had the support of a strange, brilliant doctor who'd solved the biggest mystery of my life. Well, not the biggest mystery. I was still seeking God, or something like it, but a mental health mystery that had dogged me since childhood and led to much suffering that could have been avoided if somebody had really seen me, if I hadn't been sent alone into an emotional desert by my family. I stopped at a filling station where I bought gas and a Gatorade, and then I drove the rest of the way home. I walked Blue, and then, together, we collapsed in bed.

As I drifted off to sleep, I listened to the recording I'd made of the Krishna Das workshop in Encinitas. At one point, he talked about the importance of not taking the spiritual bypass and thinking that chanting or spirituality will fix everything in our lives. "We must have courage, too," he said. "Courage to fix our lives when they need fixing." He continued, "One day when I was in India, Maharaj-ji and a few of his devotees were staying at a hotel in a distant town. Maharaj-ji was lying down. And, suddenly, without any context, he sat up straight and looked at us. He said, 'Courage is a big thing.' One of the other devotees chimed in. 'Yes, Maharaj-ji, but God takes care of us.' Maharaj-ji looked at this man, and at all of us, with piercing eyes: 'No, courage is a really big thing.'"

I had forgotten about this moment. I paused the recording, got out of bed, and walked over to the whiteboard I'd stuck to one of my kitchen cabinets. I grabbed the pen and wrote in big, bold letters: "Courage." And then I drew a big heart underneath it. The root of the word "courage," as you might know, is *cour*, "heart."

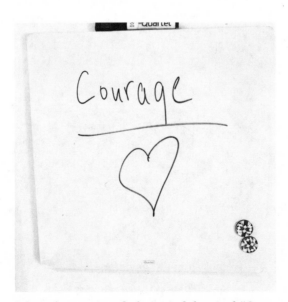

I drew this picture of a heart and the word "Courage" on the whiteboard in my cave-like studio apartment in Boulder, Colorado.

I fell back asleep, and the next morning, as I made coffee, I looked up at the whiteboard and saw the written word and the big red heart. And I remembered Maharaj-ji's words: "Courage is a really big thing."

Not a day goes by that I don't look at that same whiteboard. I haven't touched it. I never erased it, and I never will. I sometimes press my hand against it, in a declaration of the word's truth and near-physical realness to me.

Dr. Marc and his diagnosis popped, once and for all, a bubble I didn't know I'd been living in. There was now *before the trauma diagnosis* and *after the trauma diagnosis*. And I knew my task was to wake up to this healing journey with courage.

But had I forgotten about India?

No way.

twenty-three

AWAKENING

S OME MOMENTS, SOME MOODS, FEEL SO UTTERLY FULL, SO
beyond ready, as to be called pregnant—even by a childless middle-
aged man like me. Spring of 2018 was one of those times. The ship of my
life was no longer foundering. My business, though small, was growing. I
spent more time in a state of joy. I had made many new friends working
as a yoga teacher at a Boulder studio and as a yoga student in Taylor's
thriving community, a group of people like me: middle-aged folks who
saw through the pitfalls of striving for perfection and were fiercely working on loving all their messy parts.

"We are all janitors," Taylor would say at the beginning of class.
"Don't worry about making a mess. You're bound to. You're human. Just
make sure you clean up after yourself." Other days, she'd say, "If somebody hands you a flaming bag of dog shit, hand it right back to them."

For the first time since I was an editor at *Outside* in the early 1990s,
I felt part of a group of decent human beings. After yoga, we would all
wander together to the Farmers Market and drink coffee and talk about
how we could support each other. I was also in a new relationship with a
woman named Amanda. She was a tall fifty-year-old brunette who worked
as an office manager in a medium-sized advertising agency. She had two
children, a twelve-year-old boy and a nine-year-old girl, whom I hadn't
yet met but looked forward to getting to know. On our first date, Amanda
told me she suffered from a major childhood trauma. Today, I understand

better that traumatized people are drawn to other traumatized people, and that when two traumatized people come together in a romantic relationship, it can be extremely challenging. But I fell hard for her, for all the right reasons, I told myself. I'd worked hard on myself, and I believed I was ready for my forever relationship.

One morning, on my regular creek walk with Blue, I felt more attuned than usual to my natural surroundings. Over the past week or two, I noticed animals and birds that were native to the area but that I hadn't ever spotted in the previous five years: white-winged doves, turtles, a great horned owl, to name a few. These more unusual animals seemed to be everywhere we walked. The morning light seemed whiter, clearer; I swear it bent around tree canopies and buildings. Once a flock of birds formed and swirled near us, seeming to wrap us in a blanket of wings. The hawk on a tree by the library, which we saw once every few weeks, was now there every day. Did this have to do with Neem Karoli Baba? Was I really, truly, finally going crazy? Or was I finally just seeing?

Blue was the same, always staying so close as to hug my thigh. We were like a single organism moving through space and time. I worried about his health. When I adopted him, it was not clear how old he was. They said four, but I now suspected he was older, maybe six or seven. And he'd been through the wringer in his life. I worried I would soon lose him. Or was I feeling something else? The death of old ways of my being in the world. Old parts of me. I'd listened to Ram Dass talk about sacrifice. We must leave behind old, dead wood. We must sacrifice our need to know outcomes. We must turn our lives into a sacrifice—or a gift, if you prefer a more positive word.

I had made the down payment on a trip to northern India sponsored by an Amherst, Massachusetts–based yoga studio that offered international excursions. The trip, scheduled for October, was called Northern India Bhakti Yoga Immersion, and its itinerary included two weeks at an ashram in India's Kumaon hills that was ten miles as the crow flies from the ashram where Ram Dass and Krishna Das had been devotees of Neem Karoli Baba. Amanda asked to go, too, which excited me. When she made her down payment, I was thrilled about both the trip and the relationship. Maybe it was really going somewhere.

Spring turned to summer and summer to fall. The aspen leaves turned bright gold. Boulder Creek ran shallow and clear. There was just one problem: Amanda and I were not getting along. Every morning before dawn, I read the Bhagavad Gita and tried to chant it in Sanskrit. I kept circling back to the third chapter when Krishna explains to Arjuna the need to act, to bypass our neuroses, and step into our dharma, our purpose, our path. At the same time, I felt helpless in my relationship with Amanda. I had a feeling, such a familiar feeling, that it was ending. And there was nothing I could do about it. I guess it just wasn't meant to be. I'd become so consumed by my spiritual seeking that I lost interest in physical intimacy. And this infuriated her. She sat on the bed waiting for me to have sex, while I sat meditating or watching a documentary about yoga or some great Indian saint.

Looking back, I had become a little too enthusiastic about my spiritual journey. All my libido was channeled into that. I had arrived in what felt like the most important weeks of my life: a place of preparation for a life-changing trip. All summer I'd been gripped by anxiety, but instead of making it wrong and wishing that it would leave, I welcomed it. I knew it for what it was now: the old trauma just washing its way through my system. What did the anxiety have to say to me? I didn't understand it. And maybe I couldn't understand it. Was I anxious because I was going to die in a fiery plane crash on the way to India? That crossed my mind. But I suspected it had more to do with another type of death: the good old ego death. The anxiety was anticipation. Was I about to become enlightened like a great saint or guru? I doubted that, too. But I did wonder whether some part of me was indeed going to die in India. Some part of myself that needed to go. *Bring it on*, I said to myself.

The months of anxiety leading up to the India trip had cut into my business success. I had built my bank account up to about $15,000. But prepping for India cut into my focus and work hours. Now I was down to $8,000, even though I'd been driving my ass off for Uber the past month.

I heard that Boulder was overrun with drivers, and so all of us were making less money.

Amanda came over the night before our flight, and we fought again. Once again, I wasn't interested in sex, but I thought she'd understand tonight. I thought she'd be busy getting her things together for the trip. How could I have sex? I was aligning with the divine.

And I was worried that I'd have a panic attack on the plane, like in the old days. Or that I'd feel isolated in the Himalayas and my old fear of nature would kick in. After a decade of traveling the world, pushing myself alone into exotic places, I still was afraid, and I was trying to keep a lid on it. The words of one of Dylan's songs kept circling through my brain: *It's not dark yet but it's gettin' there.*

Two polarities were pulling apart inside me: on the one hand, anticipation, fullness, the possibility of spiritual awakening, and on the other, fear, death, the unknown. I feared I couldn't hold it all inside. If the time were pregnant, what was going to be born? Would I return too different to even recognize myself? Or, perhaps worse, would I return home the same man, and this entire journey would be for naught?

We threw the bags by the door. Amanda stayed back while I took Blue out for one final spin down Pearl Street. We passed a corner and turned to find a rainbow arching over Pearl Street. Jung described the difference between *coincidence* and *synchronicity*: synchronicity is meaningful. This certainly felt like a meaningful moment. Was I pulling these natural occurrences out of the ocean like Nainoa Thompson? Or were they purely coincidental?

We Ubered out to the Denver airport and took off for Frankfurt. In Frankfurt, we boarded the flight to Delhi. There were other members of our group on the flight, and we chatted back in the galley, trying to stay hydrated with bottles of water. Finally, bleary, on the ground in Delhi, we piled into vans. The heat was as I remembered it: like a wet blanket. And somehow full of life, like we were crawling into the very flesh of one of the sacred cows grazing on the side of the road. After an hour of bumper-to-bumper, horn-honking driving, we arrived at the gate to Sri Aurobindo Ashram.

For the next three days, I meditated and went to meetings. Amanda and I passed in the hallways and slept in the same bed. But intimacy was gone. She was pissed, and I couldn't bring myself to ask what I could do. I was focused on something other than human intimacy. To a fault, I admit. Even if I had rallied for sex, we couldn't have had enough of it in three days to make up for the past two months of my balking and excuses. It didn't seem to matter that we were at an ashram where sex was discouraged. Tensions were high. So I avoided her. I walked the track in the garden, brilliant with pink-and-white lotus flowers, listening to the mews of peacocks. The ashram was on the airport flight path, and planes flew low overhead every ten minutes. I didn't care. We ate dal and rice. We practiced yoga on the rooftop. We chanted and prayed. I loved ashram life; I could do this forever, and we hadn't even left Delhi yet.

On the third morning, we gathered in the lobby and rode in buses to the train. The porter who carried my bag wore a T-shirt that read, "In the end, it's you versus you." *Wow*, I thought. *Only in India.*

The train was headed to Kathgodam, a five-and-a-half-hour journey. In my seat, I dozed and drank tea and chatted with Amanda and our new friends as we rolled past villages and small cities of brick buildings and ancient-looking mud huts. At 10 a.m., we crossed a medium-sized river. I looked at my map. The Ganges. It wasn't the big Ganges of Varanasi, but still. . . . *Holy fuck. I'm here. I'm back at the Ganges, the holiest river in the world.*

The train rolled on. More villages, more smells. And then, to the north, the landscape abruptly changed. Boulder's foothills were steep. But these rose straight up out of the plains, a wall at the edge of a field.

We detrained at Kathgodam and piled into Land Rovers that were waiting for us. The highway took us up and around steep hills, overlooking mighty rivers and waterfalls and edging past steep drop-offs. As we approached corners, the driver pressed on the horn, warning any traffic on the other side that we were coming through no matter what. As was the case during my travel writing years, I felt perfectly calm. I was never scared during dangerous activities. I'd paraglided off Aspen mountain and helicoptered over Greenland. Not once had I felt fear, but the opposite. Now, I know myself: when I travel, when I am in motion, I am calm. When I stop and I am isolated or alone, I feel afraid.

We'd been driving for an hour and a half when the driver said we were within thirty minutes of Madhuban, our ashram, when a monkey dropped from the trees onto the highway right in front of us. I pressed my feet to the floor as if applying the brakes, but to no avail. We were barreling down on the monkey. It had silver fur and a gray face. It was tall. Almost humanoid. "Jesus!" I shouted. I braced myself for impact. We were going to kill a monkey on the drive up. How inauspicious could you get? And then, the monkey turned and seemed to look through the windshield. I know I have an active imagination, but I swear to Hanuman the monkey god that this animal and I made eye contact for a half second. And just as I braced for impact, it was gone. It leaped upward with both hands held high, grabbed a low-hanging branch, and then, with the force that no Olympic gymnast could muster, swung itself back into the canopy.

If my mood wasn't pregnant before, it was about to pop now.

The last stretch took us up and over a hill and down into a valley. We passed through the village of Ramgarh. Dogs hurried to meet us. People dodged out of the way. And then we dropped into a green valley with a small stream. We stopped, unloaded our gear, and carried it up the hill. We were at our home for the next weeks—an ashram. It was the most romantic place I'd ever set foot in, with a glass meditation hall, an outdoor dining area overlooking the drop-off to the valley, and our very own casita. Amanda and I unlocked the door to find two twin beds— fitting—and a billion-dollar view of the valley.

Over the next few days, we practiced yoga, chanted, listened to spiritual teachings, and meditated in the glass room. I sat on the roof of the world and wrote in my journal. I let myself enjoy the fruits of all my inner work. I had reached a quieter state in the last few years—I was far more subdued than during my pilgrimage to Holy Land. Sure, I had a ways to go, but I did feel how much more healed I was. And I wanted more. I was hungry for a more spiritual awakening. For more calm. In Sharon Salzberg's *Faith*, I'd read that Dipa Ma, her Indian meditation teacher, had encouraged her to "go for it" spiritually. Why not? Why limit aspiration? Don't expect to become the Buddha, she wrote, but there are far worse things to devote your energy and time to than becoming a better human through spiritual aspiration. But mostly, I'd been bitten by the bug of Neem Karoli Baba.

I couldn't wait to visit the ashram where Ram Dass and Krishna Das had met their guru and spent time with him. I had watched documentaries about them a hundred times, maybe more. I'd forced every date who stuck around to watch them, too. The universe and I were finally beginning to feel in alignment. I felt at home and in heaven. Or so it seemed. And it was about to get far more interesting.

Five days later, the bottom would drop out of my life. Everything that was dear or familiar or made sense about my life and the universe would be turned inside out.

twenty-four

LOVE

W E PARKED THE LAND ROVERS AT THE BOTTOM OF THE mountain. It took an hour to hike up to the cave, which was located near the top of a jungle-covered foothill. I suppose we were at an altitude of about ten thousand feet, but it seemed as if we were in the stratosphere. I unlaced my shoes and looked at the cave's entrance, a rectangular opening in the granite wall that appeared to lead only into darkness. *We will have to get on our knees and crawl*, I thought. I slipped off my shoes and set them on the ground behind a stone bench. I stood up and breathed in the moist jungle air. The leafy green canopy blocked all signs of the crisp blue sky. I followed six friends from the group up the trail's last ten yards toward the cave. One by one, we passed under a brass bell slung from a tree branch. I tapped my fingers against it until its ring filled the jungle air and echoed across the valley. Then I crouched on all fours. With my neck mala—a string of blood-red beads purchased the day before at a nearby Hindu temple dedicated to the monkey god Hanuman—dragging in the dirt, I crawled through the gap between two large boulders. The ground felt like sandpaper on my hands and knees. Seconds later, it was as if somebody had turned out the lights.

I squirmed along the coarse ground, waiting for my eyes to adjust to the candlelight. A strange world began to reveal itself. My eyes darted around at the cave's walls, decorated with indecipherable writing and framed pictures of Hindu gods, Krishna, Ganesh, Hanuman, and others. I spotted Ramakrishna, a nineteenth-century saint who taught bhakti yoga. The cave wasn't large—about the size of a small living room—but it was bigger than I'd imagined when my friend David, one of the retreat leaders, told me about it and the ancient yogi who lived there. "He's one hundred years old," he'd told me. I didn't believe him.

I was still breathing hard from the hour-long hike up the mountain, and my throat felt scratchy, as if I'd swallowed sand. The air was thick with smoke from incense and a small fire located near an opening at the back of the cave, where the smoke escaped. I set my gaze straight ahead. There he was. The one-hundred-year-old yogi. I didn't know his name. David called out to him. I saw that he had a wrinkled face and a long, orangish-white beard. He wore the type of orange one-piece outfit I'd seen other *sadhus* wearing in cities. He was seated by the fire, where he sat stirring the contents of an aluminum pot.

I kept crawling. I had butterflies in my stomach, and my heart beat hard against my sternum. I felt my age. I felt my knees. I felt the potential ridiculousness of it all. I remembered the weeks and months I'd spent lying on the couch. I remembered my absurd, middle-aged soak in the River Jordan and my visit with my personal Satan at the Mount of Temptation. And along with the inner critic, it was as if I could feel every seeking moment of my life entering the cave with me. I could feel every one of these memories, every one of these experiences. I could contact them all at once. And this feeling was big and noisy, and it felt nearly uncontainable.

I was at the tip of the spear of my life.

And then, the feelings subsided. And a straightforward, typically (for me) self-aggressive thought formed: *This better be good.* This visit with the yogi in the cave had better live up to its billing. This experience had better be what I am looking for. It had better feed the insatiable spiritual hunger that now lived in me like a tiger. *This fucking yogi better be fucking real*, I thought.

Why? Because if he wasn't real, if he felt at all contrived, I didn't know where to turn next. If this yogi was a sham, I'd have played my final hand. I would not be able to continue the strict diet of constant inner work. I would not be able to keep up my quest. And then what the fuck was I going to do? Get a job at a liquor store and buy a metal detector? Move to a trailer park in the Mojave Desert and spend the rest of my life binge-watching Netflix?

And as I entered the cave, and the light faded, and I felt cool air on my neck, I felt the in-betweenness. In the cool, dim, candlelit air, I became the in-betweenness. And then, with hair rising on the nape of my neck, I settled in. In Somerset Maugham's *The Razor's Edge*, one of my favorite books, Larry, the protagonist, a survivor of World War I, finds himself wandering the Himalayas seeking the wisdom of a yogi in a cave. That book instilled in me an image that I never shook, even as it seemed impossible that I'd ever find myself in such a weird situation. Now I was the seeker in the cave.

Despite all the worldliness and travel street cred I'd accrued, despite all the supposed spiritual and deep personal growth work I did—the yoga, the meditation, the reading of scriptures, the therapy, the books, the tapes, the weekend retreats—nothing had prepared me for what was about to happen in the cave and over the next twenty-four hours. Absolutely fucking nothing.

David approached the old man first. He set his guitar down and took off his stocking cap with the peace insignia and then bowed until his head kissed the dirt floor. As he rose again, he moved the hair from his face. He smiled widely. Then David crawled over to the right and took a seat on a burlap sack. I watched a half-dozen of my fellow travelers follow suit. Each bowed, sat up and looked at the yogi, who gave each of them a subtle nod. Then it was my turn. Mimicking the others, I bowed until I felt my forehead touch the hard dirt floor. The ground was cool like nighttime, and I felt sharp grains of sand pressing into my skin. I reached my hands out. There was nowhere to put them and so, hesitantly, I rested them on the old man's leather shoes. I worried this was disrespectful, and then I remembered reading somewhere that that's what you're supposed to do with saints, sages, and holy men in India. Still, it felt strange, awkward even, although certainly this moment never could have been easy. But I stayed there, in what Hindus call *full pranam*, for four or five seconds. At first, I wondered how long I should stay. I'd never bowed to a yogi or a guru before. And then I tried to listen to my breath. Down there, with my head on the ground, my breath sounded loud and uneven. Then, I don't know whether I willed this or it just happened, but every muscle in my body relaxed. My breath evened out. Maybe I just thought, *Fuck it*. In any case, I surrendered. I left all of me on the dirt floor in that cave. Body, soul, heart. I suppose, on some level, I said, *Take it. All. Away*. And then, I realized I'd been down there quite a while. *I better rise*, I thought.

As I pushed my hands into the sandy floor and lifted my forehead off the ground, I felt the yogi's palm strike the crown of my head. It was harder than a tap, but not quite a forceful slap. I rose so that I was on my knees, my eyes level with his. Our eyes met. His eyes were dark brown. It was like peering into the ocean from the side of a boat. At first you see what's immediately below the surface, maybe the first two or three feet down, but then if you try to look deeper, you can't. You give up. The water is too deep, too impenetrable. I held my gaze. He kept looking into my eyes. And then I felt a tsunami of emotion well up from my pelvis. It passed underneath my belly and rose through my solar plexus. It filled my chest and wrapped around my heart. And then it kept rising, up through my neck, jaw, sinuses, and, when it reached my eyes, I began to cry. I kept looking into his eyes. The wave of emotion rose into my skull all the way to the crown. Weeping. And then, he nodded. I was dismissed.

Fuck, I thought. *What just happened?*

Stunned, overwhelmed, I crawled off to the side and took a seat next to David on the burlap sack. I was embarrassed by the intensity of my sobs but felt powerless to stop them. I covered my face with my hands. Occasionally, I peered through the cracks in my fingers and looked at the yogi, who kept stirring the contents of the pot.

The next twenty minutes are a blur. The tears flowed like never before. They flowed like they'd flowed when Dr. Marc told me I had PTSD. I didn't dare move my hands away. I felt too embarrassed, given that I'd

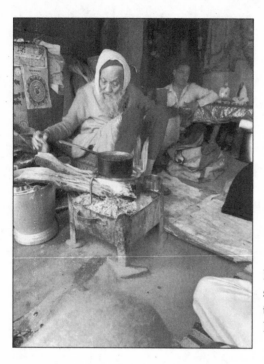

I stopped crying long enough to snap this picture of Baba-ji making tea in his mountaintop cave near Kainchi, Uttarakhand, India.

only known the members of my group for a few days. But, as much as I wanted the embarrassment to ease, I didn't want the crying to stop. It felt so good, like the tears were from decades ago. I feared that trying to stop them would risk stopping them forever, and they felt like they needed to come out. And if they didn't come out now, they might never. And I might lose my one chance to finally feel healed. As it happened, there was no stopping them. I couldn't have if I'd tried. And like a scene in a disaster movie, a dam had burst, and the head of the water board and the mayor of the town at the foot of the canyon were helpless to stop the wall of water. Nature was in charge. It was what it was.

As I wept, I heard Narendra, a local man who had agreed to guide us to Baba-ji's cave and serve as translator, talking to my friends in English. He was explaining that the yogi, whose name was Kasernath Baba-ji, had spent twenty years living alone in this cave. He was a *sadhu*, a yogi ascetic. When he was younger, he'd been in the military. But when he reached middle age, he had a conversion or transformation. He'd met Neem Karoli Baba, or Maharaj-ji. Maharaj-ji changed Baba-ji's life with his yogic teaching, similar to how he changed Ram Dass's and Krishna Das's lives. Actually, Maharaj-ji didn't do much teaching. He spoke in riddles. He playfully threw bananas at his devotees. He fed them massive quantities of food. He repeated this phrase: "Love everybody, feed people, and remember God." It was his loving presence, not his words, that his followers say was so powerful. Unlike other Hindu sages, who had complex teachings, Maharaj-ji didn't offer a method. He simply loved you. And you felt it. Apparently, in his company, you felt intoxicated with love. In recorded interviews, I've heard his followers say things like, "He loved you from the inside out." In recent years, people have postulated that Baba-ji had an abundance of mirror neurons, a preverbal system that links mammals together "brain to brain."

Baba-ji wandered as a *sadhu* for twenty-five years. And then he retreated to the cave we were sitting in now, where he'd been since he was seventy-five. Narendra pointed to a date scrawled in ink on the wall. 1995. In 1995, at seventy-five years old, Baba-ji moved into the cave. He was seventy-five then . . . I did some quick math. 1995 seemed like a lifetime ago. I was twenty-nine years old and bugging my boss Mark Bryant to let me assign the Everest story. I was a newlywed, in love with my grad school sweetheart and planning my future as an adventure writer. The world seemed like it was my oyster. This made the yogi ninety-eight years old.

Holy fuck.

I thought the crying was easing, but it welled up again as if another dam, behind the one that had already burst, had given way. And my body shook. *Jesus, what's wrong with you? Pull it together.*

I couldn't.

Had my life been leading me to this point? From editor to adventure journalist to homebound, drugged-up invalid to junk dealer to yoga teacher sobbing at the feet of a holy man? To this cave in the Himalayas? Who was writing this script?

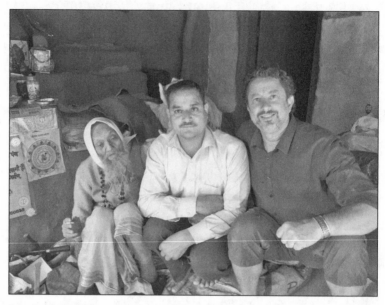

Posing with Baba-ji and Narendra Singh Mehra, my guide and translator, during my second visit to the cave.

The crying let up and my mind began to wander. I tried to imagine what it would be like living in a cave like this for a quarter century. What would it be like to meditate, chant, and pray all day? One would finally figure out a lot of shit in here. India's Himalayan foothills and their caves are a famous refuge for yogi ascetics. The idea is to deny comforts, simplify one's life, and distill or purify the mind into its essence. This is the path to enlightenment. The yoga texts call the purification process *tapas*, technically "heat" or "discipline." By sitting in life's discomfort for long periods, you burn away dysfunctional patterns of conditioning. You sit in the fury and flames of the conditioned, ever-busy monkey-mind, and eventually, it all burns off, and you are left with . . . yourself. As you indeed are. I didn't care about achieving Buddhahood, full-blown purified Shiva mind. I would have been happy with reduced suffering. I only wanted to sweep out the dark corners of my heart.

Something about the cave, and the yogi, felt familiar. Months later, I understood why. As far-fetched as it might seem, Baba-ji reminded me of me. I realized I too had been living in a cave. Admittedly, my studio in Boulder was luxurious by yogi standards. And I left my studio-cave plenty. I drove to Denver a few times a week to teach writing. I met friends for coffee. I went on dates. All of which was, admittedly, a far cry from a yogi in a cave. But I also spent an awful lot of time alone, especially compared to most Americans. Some weeks I saw no one except the people I passed on my morning walks. I lived on simple meals of rice, vegetables, and the occasional fruit smoothie. I got rid of my TV, including Netflix. I dedicated most nonworking hours to spiritual practices: I meditated and practiced yoga for three or four hours per day. I abandoned many of the luxuries that most Americans enjoy and consider to be essentials, like movies, vacations, hobbies. In my studio-cave, I read a lot of books about yoga and Buddhism, and I sat in the discomfort that thinking about my earlier life brought up for me. The memories of my family. The trials and tribulations of life. Loss. Lies. Hiding. In my tiny, cave-like studio apartment, and in the inner cave of my mind, I had been sitting with these things for quite some time. And love. Love was starting to emerge in the cave of my heart, just like it had for Ram Dass, Krishna Das, and this man here, Baba-ji.

My new friends were speaking with Baba-ji through Narendra. Katey, a seventy-ish yoga teacher from southern Indiana with whom I felt a bond, asked Narendra to ask Baba-ji about the spirit of her recently deceased mother. Narendra, speaking in Hindi, asked. By now, the tea in the pot was steeped, and the air in the cave smelled sweetly pungent. I could see the yogi forming his thoughts as he passed out cups of tea. Then he answered in long, flowing, Hindi sentences. Narendra listened, nodding. And when was finished, he turned to Katey and related to her what said. "Your mother is at peace now. It's time for you to focus on your life." Katie nodded her head and cried. She looked awestruck, relieved. I could tell that she too needed peace.

Baba-ji reached into a cabinet and brought out nuts. He prepared a tray and began passing them out. Meanwhile, Gabe, a heavyset Latino man from LA, was asking his question. "Alcohol has had a negative effect on my family and me. I'm wondering if I should give it up." His question felt close to home for me—obvious, too. But I kept listening. As the nuts were passed around, Narendra asked Gabe's question of Baba-ji, and Baba-ji paused, considered his answer, and then answered. "Yes, it's time. No more alcohol. Focus on the positive with your family."

We ate nuts, drank tea, and asked questions. Then it was my turn.

There were so many questions that I wanted to ask. I wished I could be alone with him. So many questions. And after receiving what Indians call the "glance of mercy," I felt silly asking a question in this group format. For God's sake, he was a yogi, an ascetic meditator, not a fortune teller. I ended up blurting out a question that he couldn't possibly answer.

"Should I try to rebuild my writing career or follow the path of teaching yoga and maybe teaching meditation someday?"

"Yes," he said. "I should think both."

It made sense. I nodded, yes. But I didn't really listen or even care about his answer. I was still thinking about his eyes and still feeling the impact of his glance of mercy.

Baba-ji passed the tray again. I chewed on the bland nuts and on his answer for a while. We chanted to Ram, Krishna and Radha, and Shiva in Sanskrit. I wondered how long we'd been there. I guessed three or four hours. Narendra informed us that our time was up. Our small group posed for pictures with Baba-ji. And then, one by one, we turned to crawl back through the cave's opening. I left last. I made prayer hands and bowed to Baba-ji. I thanked him. As I turned away, I felt a tug on my shirt. It was Narendra. "He said come back."

I nodded. "Yes, I will."

Outside the cave, the sunlight hurt my eyes. I slipped my running shoes back on and followed the others back down the steep trail for the long walk back to our cars. My eye caught a high tree branch swaying. I looked up and saw three or four large Hanuman monkeys moving swiftly across the canopy, swinging from branch to branch, an image of power, grace, and ease.

We rode in silence on double-track dirt roads alongside thousand-foot drop-offs back to the ashram. Overhead, more Hanuman monkeys swung on trees. In the middle of the road, dogs held their ground until the last possible second. When we arrived back at the ashram, I was still shaking my head in disbelief as I walked alone down the trail past the dining room and glass meditation room. I skulked through the fragrant flower gardens and past the lotus pond, where a single pink flower bloomed in the muck. The sun was setting, and the lush, green Himalayan foothills appeared to be wrapped in a light gauze. I kept walking until I reached the small apartment I shared with Amanda. The natural beauty and daily yoga and meditation on the trip clearly wasn't going to fix our relationship problems. I sat alone on the back porch. I wanted to think about the day. I thought I might journal about the yogi in the cave and the crying spell. But as soon as the sun went down, I felt fried. I crawled into bed and fell immediately asleep. It turned out the yogi in the cave was only the beginning. The monkey on my back—the self-doubt and loathing, the seeking, the doubting, the anger—was about to be shaken off forever.

The next morning, I woke before dawn. I snuck out of the room so as not to wake Amanda and navigated the path in the dark and cold toward a chair on a patio overlooking a steep drop-off into the valley below. I stopped in the kitchen, where I poured myself a cup of chai, and then I took a seat. I sipped my chai and read a book about yoga that I'd brought along. I was finally reading about the *niyama*, or yogic rule or observance, called *Ishvara pranidhana*, "surrender to God." It was a section I'd dismissed before. As I sat there reading, I heard a bird chirping loudly. Then a second bird. I looked up at the roof of the dining room and saw two large green birds preening each other. They seemed to be in love—partners. I grabbed my phone to take a photo of them, but they were gone. I scanned the valley and found the pair again, soaring. They soared high and far, making big sweeping loops over the valley. When they got to the slope on the other side, they swooped again, making a big looping arc and then circling back toward me. They got almost close enough for me to reach out and grab them, and then they turned again and soared back out over the valley. Out, out, out, out they flew, making several tight loop-the-loops before reaching the opposite slope, and then headed back toward me. I watched, mesmerized, as they repeated this elaborate flight path six or seven times. I wondered if their skywriting formed a message for me.

Then they disappeared.

Disappointed, I stood and walked toward the kitchen for another cup of chai. I stumbled. I caught myself and tried to take another step, but I could barely stay upright. My feet felt too heavy to lift. *I must be getting sick*, I thought. I set my chai down on a table and stumbled through the garden toward my room. Barely a foot in front of me, a giant garden snake crossed the path. But something was extraordinary about this snake; in its wake, the ground squiggled and vibrated. Scratching my head, I looked toward the mountaintops across the valley—the edge of the dark-green peaks blurred into the blue sky. The whole valley vibrated.

Back in our room, Amanda lay awake in bed. I told her about the birds and my heavy legs, the snake, and the vibrating ground. I felt paranoid. "I think somebody slipped me acid." I was grasping for an explanation. I was having a terrifying embodied experience that felt also out of my body, out of time.

"I don't know what to say," she said. "Tell me more." She sat up in bed, looking irritated. In those days, she seemed to wake up already upset at me. On some level, I knew that as a couple we were fucked. It was hopeless. I refused to give up. I did love her. But as strong as my love was this: I did not want to be single again. I feared the loneliness that I knew would set in.

"I'm tripping my balls off. The mountains and sky are blended. The earth is vibrating, even the monkeys and snakes. What's wrong with me? It's too big to describe. Sweetie, I have to keep walking. I want to find those birds again. It's like they cast a spell on me."

I opened my shower kit and instinctively looked for my old bottles of pills. My first thought was to medicate this situation. I heard Dr. Jerry's voice: "Did you ever feel too high?" I found a bottle of antibiotics I'd brought in case I contracted traveler's diarrhea. *I should take one*, I told myself. *I'm probably getting sick.* But I didn't listen to that voice.

I walked out of the room and returned to my bird-watching perch. But the birds were gone. The sun was up, and the entire valley appeared wrapped in gauze. A wave of emotion rose from my belly, passed up my torso into my neck and head. I burst into tears again.

I'd taken psychedelics a few times in the past, so I knew what tripping felt like. I'd also reached mildly altered states through meditation and yoga. I definitely wasn't taking drugs that day, and yet I was completely out of my mind. Inside my skull, I soared like the birds I'd seen. A voice kept repeating the phrase, "It really is all one."

This altered state of consciousness lasted all morning—and all afternoon. I sat in wonder. I wept. And then, as the sun set and the valley filled with shadows, my wild ride subsided. I eased back down, and again I was the man I knew myself to be. And yet I was finally whole and a little bit holy, like I was the man I had longed to become.

twenty-five

GRAPPLING

DURING THOSE YEARS OF INTENSE SPIRITUAL STUDY IN BOULder, I came across a story in the Upanishads, the earliest scriptures of Hinduism, written about three thousand years ago. There are a lot of father-son and teacher-student stories in the Upanishads. Of course there are; the brain is wired for stories, so wisdom has long been passed down orally, intergenerationally, relationally. One story stood out to me in particular, about a boy named Nachiketa, a precocious, earnest young man with a knack for seeing through bullshit and the sometimes dangerous habit of calling it out. The story is spare, so I'll embellish it here in the way it most speaks to me. Nachiketa's family doesn't understand him, and they are annoyed by his audacity. He's the black sheep of the family. One day, his father, a successful, wealthy businessman named Vajasravasa, announces that he intends to make a substantial spiritual offering to the gods. He will give away all his belongings to charity, and in exchange he hopes, or perhaps expects, that the gods will accept him into heaven. And so, in front of his community and with lots of pomp and circumstance, Vajasravasa gathers everything, including his cows, symbolic of both his wealth and holiness, and performs an elaborate sacred fire ritual. Nachiketa loves his father, so he watches closely, hoping all goes perfectly so that his father will achieve his goal of heaven. But as he watches, he notices that his father only brought his sickest, oldest cows to sacrifice, leaving the healthy ones behind. Feelings of concern grow within Nachiketa, and he speaks up: "What are you doing, father? Why are you playing this game? This isn't going to work. You will not be able to fool the gods."

When Vajasravasa hears his son's concern, he is annoyed. At first, he brushes him off. He doesn't even respond. Nachiketa's concern grows, and he speaks up again. "Father! This isn't going to work!" Again, he's ignored. Nachiketa is a persistent young man, and he speaks up a third time. "You will never fool the gods, Father." Once again, his concern is met with silence and a look of contempt. Nachiketa continues, "Well, father, if you're only going to give your sick cows to the gods, what do you have planned for me? Who or what are you going to give me to?"

Now Vajasravasa cannot contain his scorn for his son: "I'll tell you what I have in store for you! I give you to Death!"

Nachiketa responds the way any teenager told to go to hell would: "Okay, fine, Dad. You're on! I accept your challenge. I can't seem to learn anything from you, so I'll go see Death, and perhaps I will learn something worthwhile from him."

Nachiketa leaves his family and enters the underworld. He wanders until he comes to Death's door, and he knocks, but he finds nobody home. Nachiketa sits down and waits for three days until Death returns. Embarrassed by his rudeness, Death offers the boy three wishes. Nachiketa thinks long and hard, and then he responds:

"For my first wish, I ask my father not to be worried about me. Please, assure him that I will be okay." Death grants the boy this wish.

"For my second wish, I want to be shown all the intricacies of properly making the fire sacrifice to the gods." Death obliges and shows him the science of the fire offerings.

"And for my third wish, I want you to show me what happens after Death. Do we have a soul that goes on? Or is this physical world all there is? Do I have a soul?"

This question surprises and concerns Death, who tells the boy that providing this answer is too big a request. Death offers to give him instead anything he wants: money, women, fame. "Humans love this stuff," Death tells the boy. "You will love it, too!"

Nachiketa is nothing if not persistent. "Nope. I want what I asked for: What happens to the soul? What happens after we die? What is the secret of life, death, and the universe? I want to understand. I want to know what's going on in this world of human suffering and decay."

Death sees now that the boy will not be deterred, that he is sincere and worthy of answers.

In the Upanishads, this is where the story ends. The text continues with straightforward teachings that would go on to form the basis of Indian spirituality. I see this story as a celebration of the innocent, wise child in all of us who sees through the hypocrisy of the world and wishes it were different, the part of us that wants, craves, to understand the mystery, the soul within us that knows we are not our traumas, the part that longs to be free and is willing to do almost anything to get there. The part that won't stop asking for the answers. Even if it means facing Death itself or the death of all we thought we knew about ourselves and this world.

Weeks after my return from India, back in Boulder, I experienced a few episodes of similarly trippy feelings and visions as I resumed my morning walks along the river. I struggled to understand them. I struggled with how many questions I was holding, while my hands were empty of answers. How was I to understand what had happened to me in India? I knew that trauma occurs when a person experiences something too horrible or confusing for the brain to process it in the usual, orderly way. But what do you call it when a person experiences something too overwhelmingly good and beautiful to process? What happened in India was real, right?

I tried to share the details of my mystical experience with friends, with mixed results. Some things are too hard to explain. And even good friends can struggle to stay present as a fifty-year-old man prattles on about his ashram revelation. At the same time, I didn't want to hear their

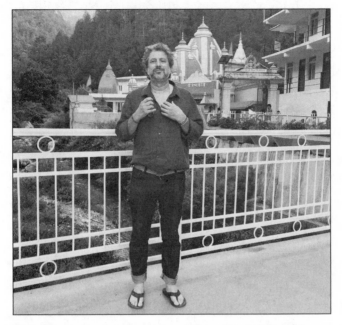

Feeling ecstatic during a visit to Neem Karoli Baba Ashram, Kainchi Dahm, India.

opinions. That day was too sacred to me. And most people are like me. We've all become doubtful and practical about life's mysteries.

Then one day, soon after my return, as I was practicing yoga on my mat in the space created by moving my coffee table, I caught myself. By searching for answers in books, I was degrading a beautiful experience by turning it into an idea—something to figure out. Something I was hoping someone else—a friend, a book, a scientist—could justify for me. If I had encountered God, why pathologize or diminish it with overthinking? *Can't you just let it be, Brad?!*

The problem was when I let it be, all I could do was cry. If I'd seen God, or even if he had just knocked on the door of my perception, I was unprepared for the effects. Over the following weeks, as I let go of trying to understand what had happened, I was a big ball of emotions that swept me into a ceaseless kind of watery fullness. It was the feeling of Everything. Sort of like the feeling I'd had at the crack in the Church of the Holy Sepulchre but times a thousand. No, a million. I'd enter coffee shops and restaurants or be driving for Uber, and these feelings would return—like my chest had been ripped open and my bloody heart was on display everywhere I went. I often thought of the massive, single tear that flowed from my mother's prosthetic eye as she had tried and failed to take one more breath. I remembered Steve Jobs's final words: "Wow. Wow. Wow." Did they experience something like what I had? Was the veil pulled back, so that they finally, truly, saw themselves and their spark merging with the great fire of life? Only my mother, Jobs, and countless others who've had such experiences were released into Death; like Nachiketa, I still had to figure out how to live.

I spent Christmas morning with Amanda and her daughter, but the writing was on the wall. By New Year's Day she seemed too pissed at me for words. I wanted it to end, too, but I felt scared that the Abyss would return once I found myself alone again. I knew I needed more help; this was trauma.

I made a few phone calls and got the name of Susan Aposhyan, a renowned trauma-focused therapist, author, Buddhist, and teacher of embodied spirituality. She had been a student of Chogyam Trungpa Rinpoche, a famous and controversial Tibetan meditation master and teacher who founded Boulder's Naropa University and coined the term "crazy wisdom." Susan agreed to take me on as a client. I didn't know what I was getting into, but I had that tight feeling in my stomach that told me this would be a ride.

When I arrived at Susan's office, I noted with relief that she had no couch, no chair, and none of the Pottery Barn decor typical of most therapists' offices. There was a futon on the floor and several cushions. I took a seat cross-legged on the futon. She invited me to make myself more comfortable. I grabbed three pillows. I sat on one and placed one under each knee. She asked me to take a breath and close my eyes. When I opened them, we made eye contact, and before I could say a word or tell a story, I was crying. I felt a sense of arrival like I'd felt with Baba-ji. I thought she was actually looking at my soul.

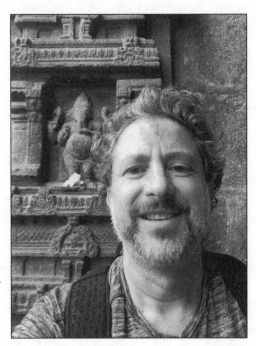

I took this selfie in Tiruvannamalai, India. The sculpture behind me is of Ganesh, the half-elephant, half-man deity in Hinduism.

After that session, I thought hard about how drawn I'd been to Ram Dass, Krishna Das, the ancient texts of yoga and Buddhism, to Jesus. What was the thread? What did all the writings and stories have in common? Soul. The river of the soul had been everywhere, the whole time, drawing me toward it, into it.

Jesus gave up his soul on Golgotha.

Yogis talked about the human soul, *atman* and the soul of all beings, the soul of the Universe, *par atman*.

Maharaj-ji, as a dead guru, was now said to be disembodied but in his Big Form, his soul form.

I ask it again, Was I seeking Maharaj-ji, or was Maharaj-ji seeking me? *Was I seeking my soul, or was my soul seeking me?*

My life journey took me to the most soulful places on the planet. We inhabitants of the twenty-first century have clouded our minds by accepting a purely materialistic worldview that has tinted the lens itself. Religious people, with their literal, dogmatic notion of faith, seem equally deluded. We have lost the ability to see the mystery. While planning for my 1997 Greenland trip, my first big adventure story mission abroad, I came across a term geologists use to describe how large landmasses that have been depressed, pushed downward by colossal ice sheets, rise again when the ice melts. The process can take millennia, but it's already happening underneath Greenland as the Icecap melts. The term "isostatic rebound" didn't mean much to my thirty-three-year-old brain, probably because I was too depressed and I couldn't imagine *not* being depressed. But as I returned from the October 2018 trip to India, the term came back to me: I was experiencing *an isostatic rebound* inside my being, in my soul. The ice of my thoughts was melting; my soul itself was rising, emerging.

Twice a week, I made my way to Susan's office and practiced.

"Brad, the good news is, you got out of childhood with your soul. That may not be true for your siblings. I'm sorry, but this work to heal yourself won't be easy. You will have to turn your life, every day, every moment, into yoga," she said.

She then gave me specific instructions in how to begin to do this.

"When you feel the Abyss, stand up and squat. Feel the weight of your legs, your hips. Feel your feet against the floor. Feel how real and solid you are. Feel that you are more than your thinking brain."

I did as she said. The Abyss still reared its head, but it held less power over me.

LATER, SHE CONFIRMED WHAT DR. MARC HAD SAID. I WAS SUFFERING from trauma—acute trauma from the canoeing accident, but also relational or attachment trauma from growing up in a dysfunctional family. Eventually, she gave me a methodology that would help me be with my intense emotions but not be overwhelmed by them.

First, she told me to say to myself, "Forgive yourself for your old dysfunctional behaviors. For the suffering you've caused for yourself and others. It wasn't your fault." She later explained that, yes, we must take full responsibility for ourselves. But the first step to recovery is self-forgiveness. She elaborated that I'd developed these patterns and behaviors unconsciously in childhood to protect myself. But now these patterns were dysfunctional, and I must adapt. Second, I was to feel the feelings, and stay present to them and to this moment by focusing on my breath or where in my body the feelings existed. I later understood this to mean that I should keep one "foot" of my mind in the memory and one "foot" in the present moment. This dual perspective prevents a person from being overwhelmed by the feelings. It reminds us that we are not actually reliving the difficult experience that caused these feelings to get stuck in the body. "You are not reliving the past," she told me. "You are safe now."

Then third, she advised me to bring some divine energy into this moment. "Think about Neem Karoli Baba, or Baba-ji, or Blue."

By staying present to this moment and the difficult feeling, I was accessing the old circuitry where the Abyss lived. By bringing the divine to it, I was helping to calm and rewire the circuitry in the face of the Abyss. "This is possible," she said. "It's not New Age; it's Buddhism, psychology, and brain science."

Around this time, I also began practicing a form of Buddhist meditation called Metta, or loving-kindness meditation. According to tradition, the practice was developed by the Buddha and given to monks living in wild, remote places in India who lived in fear of forest demons, tigers, and other dangers in the dark jungle. The practice involves wishing happiness, wellness, and freedom for oneself, one's circle of friends, one's enemies, and, finally, all the beings of the universe. The practice goes something like this:

May I be filled with loving-kindness.
May I be safe from internal and external dangers.
May I be well in body and mind.
May I be peaceful.
May I be happy, truly happy. And free.

And when you are finished with this, in a sequence of expansion, you repeat these phrases, but this time replacing "I" with names of close friends, then your enemies or difficult people, and finally, "all beings."

My "enemies" were, first and foremost, my inner critic, who I now understood to be causing my depression. He was like mud on glasses, obscuring my ability to hold my gaze, see my soul, and keep faith in front of me. Repeatedly wishing happiness and freedom for all beings trains our brain to focus less on ourselves and our own suffering and to be more available for others.

I practiced Metta for twenty minutes twice per day. I still do.

Thanks to Susan, I now had tangible tools to use, day in and day out. When I was angry at a betrayal or self-betrayal, I stopped everything and did Metta, saying the lines in full in my mind or out loud if I was alone. If a client refused to pay a bill on time, I did Metta. If I got worried about my bank account, I did Metta. If I had a triggering memory, I did Metta. I kept up with my usual tasks of writing, coaching, editing, and driving Uber and Lyft, but I also continued in therapy, practiced yoga every morning, and meditated every day. Just as there's no standard route to your soul, there is no easy path for silencing your inner critic. Just like ending any enmeshed, abusive, and decades-long relationship takes a lot of time, so does breaking up with your inner critic.

And just as I did on the yoga mat, when I lost myself, I would gently remind myself to return home. When the inner critic reared his head, I would come back to my breath, feel my body, and connect with the inner light I saw during my blow-out mystical experience in the Himalayas. This was to be my life's work. This was self-love. And when we love ourselves fully and completely, we can show up for other people in our lives. If this sounds ridiculous, if it sounds like a lot of work, well, it is. Because the game is love, and, as the T-shirt of the train porter in Delhi had read: in the end, it's you versus you.

The next time I saw Dr. Marc, I felt safe telling him what happened with Baba-ji and the mystical experience. He set his pen down and listened. And I felt no ounce of doubt or shame like I had when I told Dr.

Jerry about my "little mystical experiences" as a teen. This was as real as the river current in Arkansas, as real as the log that bruised and tore my twelve-year-old torso, facts that I kept hidden in shame from my mother after my father denied that the canoeing accident happened, as real as the hundreds of hours of meditation, yoga, and therapy. As valid as my own body was beginning to feel. As real as my soul felt, emerging.

As I finished telling him about the cave, the snake, the birds, the twelve hours on the world's roof, and how the mountains and sky were knitted together, I must have concluded with a touch of habitual aw-shucks self-deprecation that contradicted the honesty and urgency of the previous ten minutes.

"Brad, that's amazing," he said.

To remind you, Dr. Marc was as old school and professional in looks, demeanor, and approach to his work as any mental health professional I'd met. He didn't market himself as an alternative, nor would I refer any person to him who couldn't handle patriarchal attitudes. And yet I'd seen him at a few kirtans in Boulder. I spotted him in the corner, waving his arms over his head. He, like me, was a walking contradiction.

"Brad, that doesn't happen to just anybody. I know I'm a physician, but the universe is far more mysterious than I understand. And the universe doesn't hand out experiences like that unless you're ready for it, unless you've . . . earned it. You deserve this experience. I know it was real."

In mid-January, I talked with Matthew, the yoga teacher who led our October trip to India. I told him that I'd been struggling to make sense of that trip and the breakup with Amanda. I told him about the return of the Abyss. And I told him about all the work I'd been doing with Susan, the Metta practice, and the self-love.

"Brad, I feel that your soul is being birthed," Matthew said. "You're moving through something big, maybe karmic. This is about more than your childhood, more than these specific feelings." I knew what he was saying. It reflected a more Indian attitude toward our suffering. He wasn't denying past traumas or saying they weren't real, but he suggested that I might also look at my life with a slightly different slant: for reasons beyond our comprehension, perhaps having to do with past lives, our souls choose our life paths. "Come back to India with me next month. You can pay me later. I get goose bumps thinking about you standing at the foot of Arunachala. Please consider it."

I thanked him, and we said, "I love you," as we hung up.

I knew all about Arunachala. The great Shiva Mountain is in Tiruvannamalai, in southern India's Tamil Nadu state. Tiru, as the city is called, is also home to the Sri Ramana Maharshi Ashram, named after India's greatest twentieth-century saint. I'd read his book, *Who Am I?* and remembered first reading about him as the fictional character of Sri Ganesh in high school in *The Razor's Edge*. I didn't sleep that night, imagining meditating in the caves where Ramana Maharshi meditated.

I woke early the following day and typed a one-line email to Matthew: "I'll see you in India."

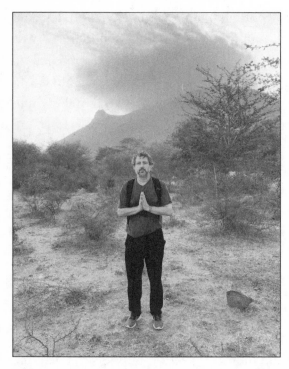

In February 2019, I stopped walking and chanting "Om Namah Shivaya" for a picture with Arunachala, the Shiva Mountain.

twenty-six

ARUNACHALA

THERE WAS NO REASON TO GO BACK TO INDIA, AT LEAST NOT now. Not four months after I returned from that magical subcontinent scratching my head and still disappearing into the ether, or the world's soul, or wherever the hell I'd been the day after Baba-ji smacked me on the crown of my head. There was every reason to stay put in Boulder and to accept his gift from the universe. Say thank you, God/universe/Brahman/Shiva, and get back to work on fixing my life. My whiteboard, which I couldn't make coffee without staring at, said it all: *Courage.* It was time to lean into courage, keep working twice a week with my trauma therapist Susan, start really building my business, and try writing again. But this time, writing articles about the topics I cared about: psychology, spirituality, yoga, with some more meaningful travel topics too. And continue to teach yoga simply because I loved it. I thought about the first line of Patanjali's *Yoga Sutra*: "Atha Yoga anushasanum," which means, "Now begins yoga. Yoga begins now." In other words, now is the time. Now is when our lives begin, not later. Now is what counts, and now is the rest of your life, distilled into a single moment. Stop wandering and seeking, and live, right?

But the more I thought about what Matthew said—"I get goose umps when I think about you on the pilgrimage around Arunachala"—the more I knew I must return to India. Something was there for me. Have you ever had that feeling? When logic tells you one thing, but your soul, or a feeling that feels so deep inside that you can't quite tell its source, tells you to do the opposite? I bought a ticket, and then I spent the two weeks before the trip reading about Shiva and watching documentaries about Arunachala and Sri Ramana Maharshi. I stumbled on this old Tamil saying: "To see Chidambaram, to be born at Tiruvarur, to die at Banaras or even to think of Arunachala is to be assured of Liberation."

The first three sites the speaker mentions—Chidambaram, Tiruvarur, and Banaras—are among the holiest in India. If you go there, you will receive a mighty spiritual boon. But no place on earth comes close, in holiness terms, to Arunachala. Arunachala isn't one of the countless places in India where a god, embodied as an avatar, is said to have vanquished a demon or otherwise saved the day. No. Arunachala *is* a god. And not any god. Arunachala *is* Shiva. According to legend, Shiva manifested as an infinitely tall column of pure white light here, and that white light turned to stone in the conical shape of Arunachala. To visit Arunachala is to come face to face with the Dark Lord, the God of Destruction, the Lord of Joy and Auspiciousness, the One Who Wears Snakes as Garlands, the One Who Wears a Garland of Skulls, the Guru of All, the Lord of All Gods, the Lord of All Beings. You don't have to go there to receive the spiritual boon; even just thinking about the place . . . well, it sure was doing something to me.

I loved this idea that merely the *thought* of the mountain would bring liberation, but I thought seeing it might pack a stronger punch. I had traveled the world seeking myself in remote and holy places. Now Matthew had invited me to the holiest place of all for worshippers of Shiva. No, I wasn't a worshipper of Shiva, not like the Indian *sadhus* were. I didn't wear a one-piece saffron outfit, smear myself in ashes, or have Shiva-like dreadlocks. But six years ago, while driving my pickup truck loaded down with my few belongings, I crossed a mountain pass at the New Mexico–Colorado border, and I called Shiva down from the heavens. I said a weird, awkward prayer while filled with swirling emotions that included the grief over my mother's death, the grief of decades of life lived trying to survive debilitating depressions, the loss of many important relationships with people who meant the world to me, real people I'd discarded not out of malice but out of fear, panic, confusion, trauma—I called on Shiva to do it: to shatter me, to break me down to nothing so that I could build myself back up from the bottom up. And I'd done it. Or I'd started to do it during the past six years. I did it by walking the creek with Blue, by religiously going to therapy sessions, yoga classes, and sitting on my meditation cushion. I did it by relearning how to make friends and build community. No, I wasn't done with the healing. But I was on a path. I found a road and I took it. And, perhaps most important of all, I stayed on it. I was "doing the work" of becoming a healthy human. I was doing my best at untangling the toxic masculinity within me. I still had a ways to go. Staying the course had gotten me this far, so staying home, staying away from Arunachala, seemed like the healed thing to do.

So I was puzzled by the messages I was feeling during the first week of February 2019. Five days before my plane was to take off, I totaled my car, which meant I had no way to drive Uber and supplement my editing and coaching income. The next morning, I went for my usual creek walk with Blue, and when I got back home, I couldn't feel my toes. Could they possibly have gotten frostbitten on one 45-minute walk in 27-degree weather? The next morning, I walked again, and my toes still hurt. I didn't think anything of it, though. How many winter mornings had I made the same walk? *There's nothing to worry about, Brad*, I thought, pushing away the now tangible pain that lasted all day. The next morning, I went walking again. And the following morning, too. And then, on Friday, as I Ubered to the airport to catch a flight to Frankfurt, where I'd transfer to a flight to Chennai, India, I couldn't feel my feet. On the flight to Germany, I noticed that my toes felt crunchy inside, like they were filled up with little crystals. I later learned that reduced blood flow to the extremities was a rare side effect of the ADHD medication that Dr. Marc had prescribed for me. But as I shuffled through the airport in my flip-flops, I was baffled by both my toes' sickly appearance and the throbbing pain. Clearly, I was dissociating from my body. Apparently, in my Shiva-lust, I'd forgotten all about self-care and self-love.

On the ground in Chennai, I met up with the eighteen people who comprised the group that Matthew and his wife, Corinne, were guiding. We were on a two-week Bhakti Yoga Immersion in southern India, in which we would explore the temples of Tamil Nadu and visit Sri Ramana Ashram and Arunachala in Tiruvannamalai. Surya, one of the women in our group, was a nurse. She immediately noticed that my feet and ankles were red and swollen. The following day, my entire lower leg was red and swollen. "You have sepsis, Brad," Surya said. "You need to see a doctor immediately. You don't want this going to your organs, your heart."

The next day, I saw a doctor in Auroville, an international spiritual community near Pondicherry, where we were staying. The doctor prescribed a heavy dose of antibiotics and told me to stay off my feet.

Yeah, right.

Over the next ten days, I walked barefoot, as the temple keepers requested, in a half-dozen temples in Tamil Nadu. Temples to Hanuman, Kali, Shiva, Ganesh, and, of course, Shiva. I swam in the Indian Ocean. I practiced yoga and meditated with the group in Auroville. We learned about ancient yoga texts. We chanted. I rode a bicycle to and from various activities. And then, on day ten, I climbed into a van with the rest of my group and rode four hours west to Tiruvannamalai, where we visited a half-dozen more temples. My feet ached. My jet-lagged mind spun. My emotions—my heart—felt exposed to the world. And then, we arrived at the base of Arunachala for Day 1 of our pilgrimage. On Day 1, we would hike barefoot, yes, barefoot, up Arunachala's flanks to the many caves where Ramana Maharshi had lived and meditated after arriving here in 1922 as a fully enlightened sixteen-year-old. On Day 2, we'd hike the ten miles in a circle around Arunachala's base while chanting silently, "Om Namah Shivaya." At least we'd be wearing shoes for that part.

After exploring the grounds of the ashram, I found a fountain with purified water. I filled up my water bottle and placed it in my day pack. I lifted my day pack up over my shoulder as I'd done countless times on my travels. I was thinking about Ramana Maharshi. According to the story, as a teenager he had mystical experiences that led to his awakening, or full enlightenment. He left his family and arrived by train at the base of Arunachala. Here, he lived in the caves and later in a hut. Over time, other buildings were added, including Sri Maharshi's Samadhi, or tomb, his mother's tomb, and the Nirvana Room. Thousands of pilgrims flocked here to stand in the presence of the meditation master. He taught the ancient Indian philosophy of *advaita vedanta*, often translated as "nondualism." The central idea is that one's individual consciousness and the consciousness of the universe are one in the same. *Moksha*, or liberation, can be achieved by disidentifying with the body, mind, and the notion of being a distinct "doer" through meditation and a technique called self-inquiry, asking yourself, Who am I? over and over until you realize there is no permanent "you" there except an inner witness who's watching the show of life. In this way, a seeker can connect with their true self-luminous nature, their *atman*, their witness consciousness. Sri Ramana Maharshi taught without speaking. Simply being in his presence was the teaching. A beautiful story, yes, but I couldn't help but wonder whether he'd experienced a major trauma. Had something happened to Ramana Maharshi as a boy that led to his leaving home, that led to his journey into mysticism? Had he dissociated from his body while scorpions practically ate his legs off during his years of meditating in Arunachala's caves?

I looked at my watch. Matthew said I could head up early to avoid the crowd; he understood my desire to travel solo, apart from the larger group. I felt ready, invigorated, and also in a lot of physical pain. I took off my shoes to begin walking. I looked down. All ten toes were swollen and red. The tips of three toes were black, and the necrotic flesh was sloughing off.

I'd edited stories about mountaineers losing toes to frostbite on mountain expeditions. But my questing had not been the kind that typically invites frostbite. I never thought I'd arrive at the apex of my healing journey, the climax of my seeking, with frostbitten toes. Or that I'd be treated in southern India, a land where average temperatures are in the nineties most of the year, by a doctor who'd never seen a case of frostbite in real life.

But by now, I knew in my body that life was full of contradictions. I felt excited and sad, grateful and scared. I put my hand on my heart and held it there. Susan had shown me this practice. I'd been doing it every day for a month. It wasn't a difficult practice. I could feel the nerves in my heart area almost turning on, lighting up. It was more challenging to maintain the energy and to do as she suggested: to see the world through my heart.

I took in a deep, big breath, one that rivaled the inhale I took before sinking below the surface of the Jordan River. I braced myself for the pain in my feet, and I took the first step onto the trail. "Om Namah Shi-vaya," I said silently. "Om Namah Shivaya." *I bow to Lord Shiva.* This was the traditional, prescribed mantra for pilgrims to Arunachala. And it was Baba-ji's personal instructions to me, which he stated during my second visit to his cave after the retreat was over. He'd said it would help ease my emotional windiness. I said it again. "Om Namah Shivaya." And again. "Om Namah Shivaya, Om Namah Shivaya, Om Namah Shivaya." Soon, the words flowed, as if the mantra was generating itself without my doing.

I moved along the path. It felt amazing to be back in India, and back at it, too—back to chasing, seeking, and visiting holy sites. What could I possibly still be looking for? What was left to find?

I couldn't articulate it at the time. Today, I will say that I was doing what I came to this earth to do. Some men seem intent on exploring the world. I tried that and wasn't up to the task. I wasn't steadfast enough to climb Everest, but I was steadfast enough for this: for trying to understand me, my past, my purpose. To realize that we have many ways of seeing ourselves and that the psychological perspective is only one perspective. I was more than just a traumatized, neurotic man. And yet, I wasn't able to permanently inhabit the soul perspective either. I was too tainted, too conditioned, or hadn't meditated enough yet. Despite the travel, effort, meditation, therapy, and seven years in bed, I was a spiritual greenhorn.

The muscles of devotion, or surrender, were still new. But that was my challenge. That was my Everest. To try to see me as God saw me. And maybe one day see others, even my family who'd cast me out, as God saw them. I wanted to learn from Matthew and Corinne. I wanted to feel the traditions of the people here in India. I guess, more than anything, I wanted it to be okay that maybe I would never stop seeking. The seeking was what made me. Maybe it was okay that I'd most certainly be back in some other weird, holy place—if not next month, then next year. While I had learned to see myself as a more whole and healthy man, I was never going to tame the seeker inside me.

I was making some progress on the actual path before me. I looked back down at the ashram plaza and caught my breath. Pilgrims were strolling around, walking into the meditation hall and relaxing under the trees. Beyond the ashram, on the street, rickshaws flew by, and vendors sold mala beads, framed photographs of Sri Ramana Maharshi, and ice cream. I took a big inhale and pushed off again, curling my toes up off the ground to avoid banging them against the rocks.

If I could have, I'd have looked beyond the street, back, back, back into my life. I still craved to understand how the boy from Kansas, the earnest, super-achieving student body president and Most Likely to Succeed trophy winner, had ended up on this long, circuitous path to Arunachala. But thank God I couldn't see the path here and that, in that moment, my gaze wouldn't stay in the past either. I was done revisiting it. I was on a new path. I breathed deeply again. I exhaled. "Om Namah Shivaya, Om Namah Shivaya, Om Namah Shivaya."

The trail was steep. Every ten paces there was a three-foot-wide stone carefully placed to serve as a step. And unfortunately, I banged my feet on almost every one of them. It was hard to feel the surfaces below my bare feet, because they were in so much pain. I guessed that I'd arrive at the first set of caves in fifteen minutes. Beyond that, there were other caves. The trail used to go to the top, but vandals had too, so they closed the upper stretch. We'd visit other caves on the back side and then de-scend and take a rickshaw back to the ashram. Tonight, I had arranged to stay alone in a hut away from the others, who were sleeping at a small resort. I needed time alone to digest all of this.

I heard a rustling in the trees to the left. I turned and peered through the trees. *Are you kidding me?* I said to myself. About twenty paces into the forest, I spotted a tall, skinny monkey. I looked more closely. It was a langur, the same type of monkey that our Land Rover had almost hit en route to the ashram in the Himalayas months before. A Hanuman monkey, named for the monkey god, the servant of Ram, who is said to be always turned toward God, always in service. And then I remembered something I'd learned from Matthew: Hanuman is an avatar of Shiva. *This is too wild for words*, I thought. Hanuman, the monkey god, has tremendous natural power and ability—physical, emotional, and spiritual— but is also said to be occasionally stricken by doubt. He is a Christ-like figure in this way. "When I forget who I am, I serve God. When I remember, I know I am God." Some said Neem Karoli Baba was Hanuman incarnated in human form. These monkeys are abundant in the north of India, but I had read that they are scarce in the south where we were. And who or what do you think Neem Karoli Baba's guru was? This very mountain I was climbing. Arunachala. The great Shiva Mountain. Of course, it was.

I kept staring at this monkey. He seemed old. Very thin. Maybe sick. He was trudging up the mountain on a parallel path to mine. I resumed my ascent. We seemed to walk together for the next minute or two. A man and a monkey. It seemed like we walked forever. We shared 98 percent of our DNA. That 2 percent that I had and he didn't created the big thinking brain, the cortex. Mine had been scrambled in the chaos of my youth, and, later, I'd medicated it into a waking coma, but otherwise, I had a fully functioning brain, and with that came maybe some special abilities, including my tendency to drive myself mad. I looked over to my left again. The monkey was gone. I stopped and listened, but I heard nothing at first. And then I heard a wild shaking of boughs, and I looked up to see the old, skinny monkey flying across the canopy with a power that no human has. He disappeared into the forest.

I was alone again. I walked. Twenty minutes later, I arrived at the first set of caves made famous by Ramana Maharshi. I set my bag down against a tree and walked up the steps and down a short hallway. I arrived at a small door about three feet tall framed in concrete. I got on my knees and crawled through. I found myself inside a dark and sweltering cave. Through the darkness, I spotted a ledge big enough to sit on. I folded my legs in *sukhasana*, or easy pose. I closed my eyes, and began to meditate on "Om Nama Shivaya," as Baba-ji had instructed me the previous fall. He said the chanting would bring me more ease and less mental suffering. I'd been faithfully following his advice. It wasn't hard to fall into a deep meditative trance with the cave's intense heat and darkness. I'd been sweating on the walk, and now the dripping was increasing rapidly. But this only heightened the intensity of the meditation, of my focus.

I sat. I cleared my mind. I felt the heaviness of my damp clothes. I breathed in the smells of the cave. The darkness and the heat weighed me down, pushed me down, like I was drowning again.

And then I thought of the boat containing my childhood friend Bill and his father crashing into the back of my head, a welcomed violent act that released me from the log in the middle of the Arkansas River. I thought of Ron, the leader of our Bible study group who grabbed me out of the river and placed me at the bottom of his canoe. I thought of Dee, the sweet friend and Bible study leader with whom I'd gone camping in Kansas and who listened to me patiently like a brother when I asked questions or expressed doubt about the Bible. Dee had been so kind to me, so supportive of my nascent faith, and so misunderstood by my family. I saw his warm grin. I thought of the counselors and kids at Maine's Camp Agawam, the beautiful lakeside refuge where I worked as a camp counselor for four years during college. There, I was treated with so much warmth and respect that I wondered whether these people, this place, was even real. I saw their smiling faces around the campfire at night. I saw my friends and colleagues from my early years at *Outside*, hardworking, funny, caring men and women who validated and nurtured my writing ability. Among them I saw Donovan, who became a world-traveling adventure writer and war correspondent, who developed PTSD while reporting in Iraq, suffered from alcoholism, and spent two years in prison for killing a man while driving drunk. I saw his big, warm smile and bright bespectacled eyes. Donovan wrote these words in an essay published in the spring of 2018: "As I slowly edge toward 60, with a broken family, virtually no money, nothing great in the way of work prospects and only my wits and a few friends who love me still around, I have a powerful remorse for the damage I have caused. But what I don't have—perhaps because I simply can't afford it—is self-pity. . . . But I have realized that there's some great power in being around long enough to comprehend that no matter the damage we've done, a new door will open." On July 4 of that year, Donovan died by suicide.

As I remembered Donovan, I understood that all this work I'd been doing was important, if not crucial. There weren't good options for anyone who avoids facing themselves and the reality of their lives. I wished to be in the same room with my former editor friend in some alternate universe.

I saw Andrew, another *Outside* colleague and buddy, who more than once talked me down from PTSD flashbacks and once wrote the ending for one of my stories when I was too spun out to write it myself. He was gone now too, killed by a careless motorist while he changed a bicycle tire on the side of a road.

I saw Matthew and his wife, Corinne, who nurtured my devotion and saw my soul being born when I couldn't.

I saw Baba-ji. Of course. And Neem Karoli Baba, Ram Dass, and Krishna Das, too. All of them chanting "Om Namah Shivaya."

I saw Dr. Benjamin, Dr. Marc, and my trauma therapist Susan—good healers, ethical healers.

I saw Di and Andrea and the other women I'd known who'd held me in their arms and listened to me late at night, early in the morning. Saints, I might call them.

And then I saw my family. I saw them as I knew them in my youngest years. My beautiful smiling mother, with her kind eyes and orange lipstick. My father, the handsome attorney who seemed too big and smart to be real. I saw my brother David, the disciplined athlete, and Molly, the smiling youngest of us. I saw us careering over the Rocky Mountains in a Ford station wagon, singing John Denver songs and hiking in Rocky Mountain National Park together. We were a family.

I felt love. Deep, honest, heart-bursting love for all of them.

Some other seekers entered the cave and the rustling of their packs and whispers broke my spell. I got myself together and headed back down the mountain.

After the day on Arunachala, the rest of our group gathered to watch a fire ceremony performed by two Indian shamans. But I felt like being alone. I left the ceremony and returned to my small bamboo hut, which sat on stilts. The sun was setting, and a full moon was lifting into the sky. I dropped onto my mattress, hoping for a peaceful rest. I fell asleep listening to mosquitoes bombard the window screens. The peace didn't last. Two hours later, I was awake, staring at the wood rafters. When it became clear I wasn't going back to sleep, I got up and went outside to the balcony and spread out my yoga mat. I moved through a few yoga poses in the dark. Moving my body like this clears energy trapped in my muscles and sinews. It makes me feel better—and sometimes allows me to go back to sleep.

Not tonight. After more yoga poses, I lay on my mat, lost in thought, staring across the grassy land at Arunachala. Clouds, lit by the full moon, shrouded its conical summit so that the mountain seemed to be glowing from the inside.

I sat upright to look more intently. It was an odd sight, this inner glow. Well, Shiva's appearance as a column of light was said to have created this majestic mountain I was staring at.

Shiva? Are you there? Show me the truth, Shiva. Shatter me and rebuild me. When I was finished talking to Shiva, I lay back on my yoga mat. I felt too fried to move. And maybe even tired of the seeking . . . for now. I considered retreating onto my mattress, under the covers, sleeping through the rest of the pilgrimage.

But I didn't.

I sat up again and stared at Arunachala and looked with my heart back at the catalyst for all of this: the night I put the corpse of my friend Paul in a body bag and knew that I was headed on that path if I didn't make a change. I looked with my heart at all the broken relationships around me. I witnessed with my heart my rage at my family, my work travels, my wanderings around the Holy Land.

And, in looking with my heart, I saw the love that had been there all along. The love I had for myself, the ways in which I had been trying to find myself and honor myself all along. Even the me that was a pathological seeker, especially that me, had been trying to save me.

I must have drifted back to sleep because the rickshaw driver's horn surprised me. Excited, anxious, sad, and at the same time filled with more gratitude for this life journey than seemed possible, I gathered my day pack and water bottle and descended the ladder to the dirt. I nodded hello to the driver and climbed into the back seat. We bounced down the dirt road to a paved highway that led us into downtown Tiruvannamalai and the gathering site for Day 2 of our pilgrimage. Now reconvened with my group, we began our walk, silently chanting the mantra, "Om Namah Shivaya."

The first two miles of the route took us through downtown Tiruvannamalai. Then we left the sidewalk for a single-track trail through the brushy landscape. I tried to stay centered on the mantra. It felt both monotonous and invigorating, a powerful tool. According to yoga texts, chanting a god's name silently invokes the energy of that god. Every few minutes, I took my eyes off the path and looked up at Arunachala's cloud-wrapped summit.

Like last night, the cloud formation was striking, but today it was totally different. The cloud had a brown tint and seemed to swirl around the mountain. It looked like a cloud of electrons. Was Shiva in that flurry of energy, waiting to heal or destroy me? Heal *and* destroy me. They were indistinguishable to me now.

My mind left the path and traveled back in time again. This time to my teenage years. It was obvious now why I'd been running—I was told I was someone to be ashamed of.

The final two miles of the path were on city streets. It was now daylight. Traffic was heavy. It was hard to stay with my "Om Namah Shivaya" as I dodged cars, rickshaws, and bikes. My mind stopped reminiscing and landed suddenly on surviving Indian rush hour. I was approaching Sri Ramana Maharshi Ashram again. The end of the walk. The end of two days walking on decomposing feet. The end of two days of the most important journey of my lifetime so far.

And then I was there, standing under the ashram sign. I had arrived.

I found a quiet grassy spot under a tree, and a swell of emotions rose inside me, too many to discern one from another: joy, sorrow, anger, relief, rage, and every emotion in between. Except for shame. There was no shame. I curled into a ball and cried. I cried for the great lengths I'd gone to seek answers and healing—decades of seeking fueled by pain. I cried over the human condition—we are all so precious and so confused. I also cried for happiness: I had done it, I was here, I was me.

Shiva had done what I asked. I was obliterated. At the bottom of obliteration was a kind of peace. There was no reason to run anymore. There was no flawed person to fix. No Bad Brad to run away from. No Better Brad to achieve. There was a greater sense of self underneath the sorrow that I could now access.

During those two days at Mount Arunachala, I glimpsed something I'd never seen before. At least not since I was a boy. It was only a glimpse, so I can't say for sure what I saw. But during and after my circumambulation, I peered deeper inside myself than I had before. Deeper than during the most focused yoga or meditation session. Deeper than during any adventure to a far-flung natural place. Deeper than during the most prayerful visit to a sacred site or Indian temple. Arunachala shattered me. Opened me. And through the tears, I glimpsed something bright, essential, and true. I don't know what to call it. So I'll call it my soul.

Epilogue

I T IS THREE YEARS LATER. I NOW LIVE IN AUSTIN, TEXAS. I MOVED
there a year ago for a relationship. Am I chasing again? Perhaps. I
still live alone. I still suffer debilitating emotional flashbacks, and I get
pulled back into hours-long dissociative states and can barely stay upright, though far less often than I used to. Sometimes tears flow and I
don't know why. Except that I do know why. I wonder whether I will
always need a lot of time alone, whether aloneness is my destiny. I miss
the Rocky Mountains. I feel naked without their grounding effect and
late afternoon shadows. Instead, my new home buzzes with the sound
of traffic on I-35 and the cooing of white-wing doves. These doves seem

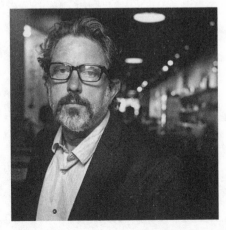

My friend, the photographer Stephen
Collector, took this picture of me shortly
after my return from Arunachala in 2019.

to be everywhere in my neighborhood, fluttering from live oak tree to Texas ash to desert willow. I do see them as a symbol, a sign that things are much better and that I'm connecting with my soul. I still can't sleep past 4:45 a.m., no matter what time I go to bed. I cherish the predawn darkness and the sound of the doves. It's still my favorite time of day.

I stumble out of bed. At fifty-six, I'm beginning to feel my age in a new way, despite daily yoga practice and swimming. My midsection is a little thicker. My knees, which have endured multiple surgeries, are arthritic. My lower back gets out of whack easily. The bottoms of my feet ache with fasciitis. I tread carefully so as not to bang my toes against corners or raised tile—they're still extremely sensitive at the site of the frostbite. But despite everything, I feel strong. Stronger than ever. In body, mind, spirit. My soul—I feel it. If you look at me today next to a picture of me from 2010 or so, you see a different person. Gone are the puffiness; the glazed, vacant eyes; the sickly, almost green tint to my skin. All those symptoms were side effects of the massive quantities of medication I took then.

I make coffee and walk toward my altar. I pass a black-and-white photograph of me taken in 1999 at the Chennakeshava Temple complex near Belur, Karnataka, India. In the photo, I am about to ascend some steps between two ancient statues of Ganesh, who sometimes places obstacles in our way, too—and enter the dark temple. The way the photograph has captured the moment, the open door to the temple is pitch black. To me, the blackness represents the dark path I was about to walk. I look okay, I was just thirty-three, but I see the heaviness and puffiness creeping in. I remember at the time feeling as I did for the first four or five decades of my life: simultaneously adolescent and ancient. I was a pathological people pleaser, but at the same time I was the opposite: rash, brash, unmoored, rebellious, and yet world weary, wise, and sage-like at the same time. Like I could hold my own playing a yogi in a mountaintop cave.

But that black door. Sometimes it scares me a little. The next two decades were going to be so challenging. Years of depression, years of extreme overmedication, years of brain fog, and then—what? A decade spent living month-to-month in a three-hundred-square-foot studio apartment, doing the hard work of reclaiming myself, my soul. I can't gaze at this picture too long because it makes me cry. I am so proud of that younger man. He did it.

I set my coffee down on the floor next to my meditation cushion and bend over to light a stick of nag champa incense. I blow out the flame, and the smoke rises, curls, moves around my altar. My living room begins to feel like that Shiva temple in Varanasi so long ago. I sit and cross my legs. I gaze at the altar, which has grown over time. The altar itself now takes up a significant part of my living room, though the top is still ringed in white Christmas lights. I look at the various objects: the old ones I placed there in 2013 when I moved to Boulder and new ones, from my travels in India and elsewhere since then. A framed picture of Sri Ramana Maharshi, the great twentieth-century saint of Arunachala, one of Sri Ramakrishna and another of Andandamayi Ma, two Indian saints whose teachings hold meaning for me. A rubber Gumby-like figurine of Jesus. A tall glass-encased religious candle with the image of Jesus on the front, ripping open his own chest to reveal his heart.

I look at a framed photograph of Neem Karoli Baba. Unshaven, wild eyed, and wrapped in a plaid blanket, he looks like he could be somebody's weird uncle. Was he working behind the scenes in my life the entire time, pulling me back to India, yanking me back into my heart? Krishna Das says that when we look at Maharaj-ji, we should remember that he is always looking at us. It's just us remembering to look back at him. I don't know whether that's true, but I like the idea of it. Some days I know it's true; other days, I think Krishna Das, and I, too, might be a little crazy. My gaze moves to the framed photograph of Baba-ji stirring a pot of tea in his cave. He looks too ancient to be real. His long, scraggly gray beard is tinted orange. His eyes, the eyes that I stared into and that stared back into my soul. They are deep, brown, seemingly bottomless. How did he know that I needed his sweet blessing—being smacked on the head? I wonder whether it was the way I held my body or the hunger in my eyes. Whatever it was, he knew. Or maybe I'm making up the story that he recognized a soul in need. Maybe he just felt like smacking somebody that day, and I was the guy.

Sitting now as I did then, I think about the twelve hours spent on the roof at the ashram in the Kumaon hills. I do not doubt that the mystical experience there was real. To me, five years later, it's as real as my coffee cup. As real as the paper on which the photo of Baba-ji is printed. It's as real as my chest feels when I place my hand on my heart.

I did honor his request to "come back" for a second visit. Narendra, Amanda, and I hiked to the top of the mountain and entered his cave a second time after the yoga retreat. I spent another afternoon with him. Again, we communicated with the help of Narendra. I told Baba-ji how conflicted I felt about my family. I loved them, and yet I knew that it was best that I take space from them. Maybe forever. I told him I felt guilty about this, and that I wanted to forgive them and forgive myself, too, for my own role in the family dysfunction that caused me so much suffering—and who knows, maybe them too? Narendra relayed my question to Baba-ji. Baba-ji nodded, and he spoke his answer to Narendra in Hindi. Baba-ji looked at me while Narendra spoke these words back to me. "It's okay, Brad. It's okay to walk away from difficult people. But remember, this is also true: You must never send them out of your heart. Keep them in your heart."

I close my eyes. I feel tears beginning to form. I breathe. Inhale. Exhale. The tears cease to form. I think about the air I breathe. Though I live in a modern apartment building, I know that the molecules of air entering my lungs are ancient, billions of years old. Odds are, this air has been breathed before by somebody, maybe countless somebodies. The rock—the calcium—that forms my bones and the water that fills each cell, each teardrop. It all belonged to many somebody elses, too. We are all ancient; at the same time we are here now. And this feels important to remember. I keep my mind close to my breath. And then I open my eyes again and look at the other photographs on my altar. One of Di, taken near our former home outside Santa Fe, one of Andrea, and one of

Madeleine, who is my girlfriend today. Madeleine and I love each other, and we both have had a difficult time understanding relationships and intimacy. We are working hard together at love. Yes, all this work can be exhausting—but what's the alternative?

There's a small open space on my altar. I think I might place a photo of my family on the altar, too, one day. Someday, I'll get around to it. It feels important to send them blessings, good energy. I hold them in my heart, even if I am not with them in person. I have done my best to let go of my resentments and to see us as friends from long ago. Nothing more. I came into this world with them. I learned much: things both useful and not. But they weren't my soul family. As Susan reminds me when I lose track, *I am a child of God now*. A child of the universe. I think about a quote from Mother Teresa: "The problem with the world is that we draw the circle of our family too small."

I return to my gaze to Baba-ji. He left the body, as the Indians say, about a year after our encounter in his cave. On a cold February morning, while I walked Boulder Creek, I received a group text from a friend in India. "I bring sad news. Baba-ji left his body last night. He was murdered by thieves." I cried with grief and rage. Who could do such a thing? And then I remember the Buddha's teachings. The brokenness of it all. The way the universe is like a new teacup, and we are to think of everything—family, dreams, ourselves—as already broken. The Japanese have made an art form of this concept: *kintsugi*, which is to mend broken teacups and other items with gold. The once-shattered cup is now repaired, with lines of bright gold illuminating the once-broken spots.

I look at a photograph of Blue. In the picture, he lies on my belly, smiling widely at the camera. Blue, the dog of my dreams, a little sausage-like being, as great a being as I've ever known, if you view greatness as the simple capacity to love. Nine months after I returned from Arunachala, on Thanksgiving Day, I came home from dinner with friends to find Blue in crisis. He was struggling to breathe and sick to his stomach. There was twelve inches of fresh snow on the ground, and the weather service advised against driving. But I knew he needed me to help him. Or, actually, he didn't. I just refused to see that his time was almost up. I picked him up in my arms and placed him in the passenger seat. I drove as fast as I could to the emergency vet. There, I set him on the floor, and lay with him, as the doctor checked his heart rate. She'd seen many dogs his age arrive in this shape, and she knew. "Blue's time has come, Brad. I think the compassionate thing would be to help him go more peacefully." She left the room, and I spent a few more minutes lying with him, stroking his gray coat, and speaking to him. I thanked him for coming into my life. For his loving presence day in and day out during the past six years when sometimes it seemed as if I had not another soul who cared about me. I now know I was wrong about that. I had more people who cared about me than I knew. I just couldn't see it through the fog and shame. And, of course, I've always had Neem Karoli Baba looking after me. He was chasing me the entire time, reminding me to love myself.

The doctor came back into the room. She stroked Blue's back and told him he was a good boy and that everything was going to be all right. She went about the task of euthanizing him, as I held him in my arms. His eyes, tired and cloudy, blinked every so often. His breath slowed. I wept. I couldn't imagine life without Blue. Sounds crazy for a fiftysome-thing man to say. But it was true. Blue opened his eyes. He closed them. "You can go now, Blue," I said. "It's okay. I'll be okay. You can return to the soul of the world. You'll be free." And then, he took one final breath, lifted his nose off the floor, and, his last act, he licked my face.

As I stare at Blue's picture, I wipe a few tears from my eyes. Blue was the best.

Last, I look at my photo of Arunachala, the great Shiva Mountain, rising from the plains of Tamil Nadu. I think about its caves and the countless "Om Namah Shivayas" I said while circumambulating. I could get lost for hours thinking about the sickly old langur, the Hanu-man monkey, who briefly became my hiking partner, or the steamy, dark caves and the powerful, laser-like meditations I had inside them, with insights into my own life I believe I couldn't have gotten anywhere but there, on the Shiva Mountain. But if I let my mind wander too long on Arunachala, it might drift back further in time to the Kumaon hills and the feeling of universal love that wrapped me up in a cosmic blanket and showed me that, I, too, was made of love, and who knows where my mind would drift from there? To the Ganges? The Chama River? Copper Canyon? The waterfalls on Greenland's Icecap? Boulder Creek? Or to the White River in Arkansas?

Come back, Brad, I say gently. Come back to this moment. You've got things to do today.

It's not easy to come back. I get stuck in the past, stuck on one word: Why? Why did it take so long to arrive here in this place and time in which I feel more solid, more content, at times almost peaceful?

I suppose the answer isn't very satisfying. I guess it just takes this long. It just does. It does because . . . we humans are so prone to running and chasing. We run away from suffering, and we run toward shiny objects that we think will help us feel better. I made the circumstances of my life worse every time I ran from myself, every time I chose running away over accepting my suffering. Every time I chose more pills over facing the truth of my life. In my twenties and thirties, I couldn't bear myself, and so the fog of the drugs stole years from my life—and kept me from maturing, too. And when I woke up from the fog in my late forties and early fifties, I found myself a grown man with the emotional windiness of a teenager. And even then, I chose to keep running—for a while longer. Every time I chased casual sex and unfulfilling relationships instead of being with myself. I ran and chased some more. Eventually, I couldn't stand myself any longer. Finally, I decided to do something about it. I did the work. And I learned to stay.

I have empathy for myself and all of us on this journey. Because chasing and running is what we humans do, especially here in the West. We chase achievement, we chase money, we chase comfort, we chase adventure, we chase, chase, chase. We run away, run away, run away. And, yes, I still do it, too. Of course I do. To live a life of no chasing would mean I was a Buddha, which I'm clearly not.

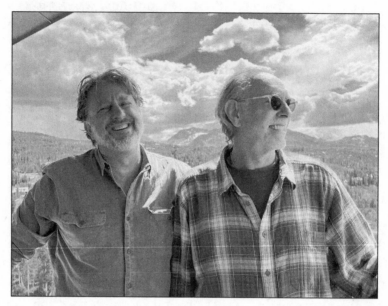

My current partner Madeleine Tilin took this picture of Krishna Das and me at a yoga festival in Telluride, Colorado, in 2022.

But I have learned to soften how I talk to myself. I have learned to catch my mind more often when it runs away from me. And that's something. In my case, it might be everything. The entire reason I feel more or less healed these days? Simply put, I accept myself more. I talk more gently to myself. Some days, I love myself.

And Baba-ji. His eyes, the twelve-hour mystical experience. The day I saw across the Universe and into my soul—into the soul of the world. I suppose you should take this with a grain of salt, because why should you trust anybody with something so profound? But I know. I saw. There is goodness in our hearts. There is peace out there, and we might only be able to taste it occasionally, but it's out there, or maybe it's in here. In our hearts. Perhaps someday we humans will see how close we are to living in peace, with less war, climate crisis, racism, and toxic politics. The ancient wisdom traditions, the great yogis of yore, said so: we can do better. Some days, I have faith that they were right. Some days it's harder to. This stuff is not easy.

I look at my watch. I'd better hurry up. I'm scheduled to teach my morning yoga class in ten minutes. Afterward, I will take my dog Tommy, whom I adopted a month after Blue died, to Barton Springs to walk along the river. Lush trees, slow-moving water. It's different from a Colorado stream. But it's becoming home. The River is still everywhere.

I take out my laptop and open Zoom. I spread out my mat on the floor. I hit Start Meeting, and my students appear on the screen. We begin. After an hour-long yoga class, the final pose is *shavasana*, corpse pose. As they lie on their backs, I tell them, "Nothing left to do. Nothing left to think." And I recite a quote that has become my mantra, my aspiration. The quote is from Neem Karoli Baba, and it goes like this:

"Why try to figure it all out when you can love."